COLLECTED WORKS OF
CHARLES BERG

IØ127835

Volume 4

THE FIRST INTERVIEW
WITH A PSYCHIATRIST

THE FIRST INTERVIEW
WITH A PSYCHIATRIST

and the Unconscious
Psychology of All Interviews

CHARLES BERG

Routledge
Taylor & Francis Group

LONDON AND NEW YORK

First published in 1955 by George Allen & Unwin Ltd

This edition first published in 2022
by Routledge
4 Park Square, Milton Park, Abingdon, Oxon OX14 4RN

and by Routledge
605 Third Avenue, New York, NY 10158

Routledge is an imprint of the Taylor & Francis Group, an informa business

© 1955 George Allen & Unwin Ltd

British Library Cataloguing in Publication Data
A catalogue record for this book is available from the British Library

ISBN: 978-1-032-16970-5 (Set)
ISBN: 978-1-003-25348-8 (Set) (ebk)
ISBN: 978-1-032-17065-7 (Volume 4) (hbk)
ISBN: 978-1-032-17116-6 (Volume 4) (pbk)
ISBN: 978-1-003-25185-9 (Volume 4) (ebk)

DOI: 10.4324/9781003251859

Publisher's Note
The publisher has gone to great lengths to ensure the quality of this reprint but points out that some imperfections in the original copies may be apparent.

Disclaimer
The publisher has made every effort to trace copyright holders and would welcome correspondence from those they have been unable to trace.

This book is a re-issue originally published in 1948. The language used is a reflection of its era and no offence is meant by the Publishers to any reader by this re-publication.

The First Interview with a Psychiatrist

AND THE
UNCONSCIOUS PSYCHOLOGY
OF ALL INTERVIEWS

BY

CHARLES BERG

M.D.(LOND.), D.P.M.
Fellow of the British Psychological Society
Consultant Psychiatrist to the British Hospital for
Functional Nervous Disorders
Late Physician to the Institute for the Scientific
Treatment of Delinquency
And to the Tavistock Clinic, London

LONDON
GEORGE ALLEN & UNWIN LTD
RUSKIN HOUSE MUSEUM STREET

*Printed in Great Britain
in* 11 *point Bell type
by C. Tinling & Co., Ltd.,
Liverpool, London and Prescot.*

INTRODUCTION

THE surface of things is often meaningless. It is only when the
unseen depths are brought to light that meaning emerges.

I have read books on the psychology of The Interview as
sterile and meaningless and dull as life itself without its hidden
meaning. A patient once told me: 'Doctor, I am dead. I feel nothing. I merely go through the motions of living.' If we only go
through the motions of living, if we see only the appearances and
feel nothing and understand nothing, we are robots. There is no
interest, no drive; the essence of life is absent.

The essence of life is the feeling of the instinct, appetite, or
lust that impels. It is the incentive behind all activity, all life; and
it alone can give us the meaning of what we do and think. It exists
unseen in the most apparently superficial human relationship,
even in the interview—as this book will show. It explains what
is otherwise meaningless.

Some may think that my case-papers over-emphasize sexuality.
That is because they are based on truth not fiction—though
identities are concealed by composite portraits. It is a fiction of
culture that sexuality is not important. More often than not
sexuality, or its apparent absence, is the corner stone of the whole
situation. At a psychiatric interview the problem presented
appears to be incomprehensible, clueless, until an insight into the
individual's sexuality knits everything together and shows the
meaning in what was previously meaningless, as the love-motif
does in Fiction.

What are the primary bases of the relationship of one person to
another? The first post-natal relationship began with an oral one
between the baby and its mother's breast. There is evidence that
the mental relationship of these two persons took its pattern from
this level, 'whole-object' and personality relationship growing,
as it were, out of what is called in psycho-analysis, 'part-object'
relationship. The result is that a need for companionship and
security appears, for a time at least if not throughout life, to take
precedence over all other personal-relationship requirements.
Finally, ontogenesis or development leads in the direction of

genital relationship, which is, of course, like the earlier mouth-breast relationship, phylogenetically entrenched.

Recently a very normal woman undergraduate said to me, in order to explain why a particular male lecturer had figured in her dream: 'I had noticed at the classes that he was *aware* of me . . . and so I had been aware of him. Nothing was said of course, but now that this dream has brought it up I realize that the situation was, and is, sexually stimulating.' Can anything be more relevant to the subject of personal relationships of which The Interview is the initial sample?

Roberta Cowell, in his description of his observations during the change from man to 'woman,' remarks that he found himself becoming progressively less interested in women, and, what is perhaps equally relevant, he found that women, strangers around him in public vehicles, and so on, were obviously becoming less interested in him. This was even before he assumed female dress. But dress too, no less than figure, acting as a fetish, can be the stimulating or suggestive factor. I remember how incensed a middle-aged gentleman became when he was told that the 'young lady' to whom he had been paying so much attention at a Fancy Dress Ball was really an adolescent male in disguise.

However, I should mention that I do not believe that *all* human relationships are overtly heterosexual or homosexual. Some appear to be based upon infant-parent or parent-infant seekings. I should add, however, that psycho-analysis, especially through a study of the perversions, has shown that even such relationships have sexuality behind them, however unconscious or 'aim-in-hibited.' The point is that there is an instinct basis at work in all cases, however much concealed. In some cases the predominating instinct drive may be that of the aggressive or destructive instinct. This could be regarded as the antithesis of sexuality.

It would tend to disrupt, or drive apart, at least in civilised communities, those reciprocally sensing such feelings, and, therefore, in the study of actual human contacts it is not so evident, except perhaps as an undercurrent or resistance. It is more liable to reveal itself by the absence of contact. Introverted and withdrawn people, people who eschew human contact, may often have an undue proportion of such repressed instinctual elements. However, they do sometimes emerge in actual personal relationships, especially in people with whom they have become an accustomed reactive pattern, ingrained in childhood. This is revealed in some of the case-papers, particularly in the latter ones. However, it seems to me personally that the so-called destructive (or death-) instinct is so largely reactive to frustration that it is difficult to extract the alleged primary factor, though I would not deny its presence.

I once saw a close-up cinematograph picture of a caterpillar's jaws lustily devouring the edge of a leaf. Was this a revelation of the aggressive, destructive instinct at work? Or was the caterpillar merely reacting aggressively (in keeping with the pleasure principle) to *frustration* (of its hunger-instinct gratification) by the *inertia* of the leaf? To me this was a picture of the *life*-instinct at work, the instinct responsible for the survival and development of the entire biosphere. It loses nothing of interest if we think of it as chemically and physically determined. Indeed, I think of the mind as a product or function of nuclear synthesis. To me, there is no break, there is a 'closed loop', a 'mechanically' or physicochemically determined *continuum* between 'primary' energy, with its nuclear forms, and the psycho-socio-biosphere.

Is the baby when sucking (or/and biting) reacting similarly to the caterpillar? Some of the later case-material may suggest that it was love-gratification that the patient (as an infant) primarily wanted, and that it was the intolerable frustration of this which led to the superabundance of anxiety, aggression, destructive impulse, hate—and illness. It is biologically and physiologically normal to fight for one's life, and every interference with gratification is physiologically and psychologically reacted to as an interference with the living process and a threat to life itself. This applies to the gratification of complicated acquired reactive patterns as well as to the gratification of instincts.

Every organism hopes that it will be loved, and its life-processes, its gratification processes, facilitated, not denied it and frustrated until it is gradually edged out of life or deprived of the desire to go on living. The infant has commonly had to give up more of its primitive gratifications than it has received compensatory gratifications on a sublimated plane. No wonder it gets ill.

Whenever an individual, overtly ill or suffering merely from civilization, meets another individual, the unspoken and usually unconscious reaction in the deeper, unseen emotional levels of the mind is this: Is this person a potential gratifier, or a frustrator and destroyer? Is he friend or foe? Seeing that we are ill through having encountered a superabundance of the latter, however consciously well-meaning, there is small wonder that most of us bring to the first interview, and thereafter to subsequent contacts, a wealth of resistances and defensive attitudes which impoverish the contact as a pleasure-giving and therapeutic experience.

The art of therapy and indeed of all human contact is to dispel these suspicions, remove these defences and supply on a mental plane what mother's love, and subsequent human contacts, should have supplied at the very beginning of life. Only then will become possible the long overdue relief of anxiety, and the relaxation essential to health and happiness. But first we should ourselves be aware of the unseen, even denied and repudiated, emotional reactions, the instinctual hopes and fears, their cause and their source; and how to expose them and how to deal appropriately with them.

CONTENTS

CONTENTS

PARTS III TO V: PRACTICE

PARTS I AND II: THEORY

PART ONE

THE INTERVIEW

CHAPTER I

PLAN OF THE BOOK

THE object of this book is to convey to the reader what every analyst knows to be true, namely that the interview, any interview, every interview, is not simply what it appears to be on the surface. Its essence will be shown to be something deeply emotional and mostly unconscious. I would not say that there is *no* connection between the conscious superficial aspects of the interview and the largely unconscious emotional reactions which accompany them, but the former are often a very poor clue to the latter; indeed, the conscious activities may be specifically designed to cover, to hide, or even to contradict what is going on unconsciously. We shall see that this is largely because we are all childishly and unnecessarily frightened of what we are endeavouring to control and hide, even from ourselves.

Further, I hope to show that it is the neglected or disregarded aspects of the interview that usually determine its effects and consequences, that *matter* far more than anything of which the parties are conscious. More than this, I hope to be able to demonstrate the nature of these unseen emotional actions and reactions, in general and in some particular instances.

I trust that this will not prove an idle study. I believe that it will not only enlighten the reader, giving him an insight into things of which he previously had no conception, but that it will put him in a position to direct his relationships to other people in accordance with his emotional purpose, or in accordance with his reality purpose, and give him at least an inkling of the ability and power which can usually be obtained only by subjecting oneself to a protracted course of analysis.

Finally, I hope to show that the subject matter of The Interview is as large as life itself. It is an epitome of every human relationship, and of human relationships in general. It will be seen, in the later chapters, to be concerned with the deepest levels of our emotional life, including those of the instincts which ensure our survival and that of our species.

However, before I can hope to bring these fundamental matters to the recognition and appreciation of everyone, I have naturally to proceed from the surface. I must utilize that which is already conscious and recognizable to lead us to a recognition of the resistances which hide from us those deeper levels of which we are so much, and so unnecessarily, afraid.

I propose, therefore, to use simple non-technical language, even when describing medical, psychological, and analytical interviews in order to make the subject matter useful to everybody, for I hope that at this stage, that of the first interview, everybody may be able to understand the unseen implications of personal contact.

Therefore, I shall begin at the most conscious and obvious surface of things, with little more than a hint that there is something more going on than would appear to be the case. I shall then have to yield some tribute to such various factors as the conscious purpose for which the interview occurs, admitting that the conscious purpose may, in some circumstances, appear more or less to vitiate some of my implications. Nevertheless, it will be shown that the general principles developed in connection with medical and analytical interviews are applicable, with modification, to practically all interviews.

A further aspect of the subject that will have to be taken into consideration is the difference in psychological reaction between interviewer and interviewed. This difference may prove important enough to justify a division of the book into two parts, so that we can study the psychological reactions of the interviewer separately from those of the interviewed.

Even from the point of view of the interviewer alone there will be differences determined by the purpose, if any, for which the interview is taking place. Naturally, the interviewer's unconscious, as well as his conscious, reactions will be much influenced by the purpose, nature, or type, of the interview he is conducting. Nevertheless, it will be seen that at the deeper level there is usually something in common despite these great superficial differences.

To underline the matter, I shall survey briefly a variety of interviews with which I am familiar, according to their purpose; such, for instance, as the ordinary doctor's interview with a new patient, the psychiatrist's diagnostic interview, the therapeutic or healing interview, and the analytical interview, that is to say, an interview arranged with the prospect of conducting a psychological analysis. I shall have to give examples of these because it will be appreciated that, in some respects, there are as many different techniques of first interviews as there are different patients and different people.

I do not think I shall be able to say much, if anything, about interviews which are not in the general run of my daily occupation, such as interviews connected with applications for employment, salesmanship, showing oneself off to advantage, the actor's or artist's 'interview' with his audience or with different types of audience, and so on. But I do believe that the knowledge we shall gain from our study, particularly our study of analytical interviews, will throw some light upon the nature of all interviews, and may even be of assistance in relieving us of anxiety in connection with them, and, through insight, may enable us to handle them more appropriately.

After this general survey, I hope to be able to expound some of the unconscious factors common to all interviews. I shall then proceed to a discussion of the psychopathology, that is to say, the morbid elements, conflicts, and complexes which affect even the most normal amongst us to such a degree as to inhibit or even to vitiate our freedom and intellectual ability to make the best of ourselves.

If, after this, I have sufficient space at my disposal, I may touch, in a superficial or popular way, upon what could be regarded as the protracted or *continuous interview*—a term which I am here using as a synonym for psychological analysis. There is some justification for the use of such a concept in that the first analytical interview is rightly regarded as epitomizing, in a superficial way, the technique or process of what may become a complete analysis.

For the second portion of this book I have the idea of giving examples of case material of patients' first interviews. If it is considered advisable to pursue this subject any more deeply, I may give some examples of the essence of analytical work in the form of case material representing the transference stage of analysis, (Part V), its handling, and its interpretation.

Finally, I am hoping that I may have space to interpose a few brief notes on the philosophy of psychological analysis, and of psychology in general, anticipating that the path will be cleared for this by a demonstration of the abundance of unseen activity that goes on in the emotional levels of the unconscious mind, even during such an apparently superficial personal contact as that of the interview.

As it is unlikely that I shall be able to cover every aspect of my subject, I propose to concern myself more especially with what I regard as the essence of the matter, namely, as I have said, that aspect of the interview which is almost universally neglected, ignored, or unseen—the stone neglected by the builders—for, without a recognition of that aspect, human relationships, and indeed life itself, remain meaningless. I hope that this unseen factor will be recognized as fundamental to the structure of interviews of every variety and pattern. The most difficult part of my task will be to make the reader see and appreciate the importance of this basic matter clearly and vividly enough for him to be able to use it himself.

I believe that I have the highest authority for my general point of view, for recently several eminent psycho-analysts appear to have been heralding a change in analytical orientation. The 'Annual Survey of Psycho-Analysis' has recently drawn attention to this. In furtherance, if not in contradistinction, to previously held views, such as those concerned with the development of instincts, the concept of what is called 'object relations' now occupies the foreground in importance. ('Annual Survey of Psycho-Analysis', Vol. I, page 230.)

The most important field for investigation of this coming theory is said to be the analyst's relation to his patient, and its implications. This is entirely in keeping with what has been recognized in the practical, clinical, or technical field of psycho-analysis, namely that the *transference*—that is to say, the patient's emotional relationship to the analyst—and its interpretation are the essence of psycho-analysis.

After speaking of the opening stage of analysis and referring to the 'inexperienced analyst', I once wrote: 'Where he is likely to fail will be at the following or transference stage, but I am afraid failure *there* will, in the psycho-analytical sense, be fundamental.' ('Clinical Psychology', page 367). This opinion still holds, but I have had some cause to revise my previous remark about the interview and the first stage of analysis. I wrote: 'Even the inexperienced analyst may manage this stage with some degree of success, provided he is sufficiently passive, and shows no affective re-action.' However, I am now hoping that, with adequate under-standing of this book, my statement may approximate to the truth, at least as regards the handling of a first interview.

It will be seen that one of the reasons for selecting the interview for special description is that, without a personal analysis, readers are not likely to benefit by a similar detailed exposition of the *subsequent stages* of an analysis. It may be doubted whether, without a personal analysis, the average intelligent person will be able adequately to understand all the fuss I am making about such an ordinary matter as an interview, or talk, with another person, but I think that at least something will be gleaned, whereas in similar treatment of the more advanced stages of analysis there lies the danger that more will be misunderstood than will be understood. Therefore, let us be content to concentrate upon the initial, open-ing phase.

The reactions of patients and the policy to be pursued with them are only special instances of the reactions of all persons everywhere; and if we would win people, if we would win their transference, if we would 'make friends and influence people', this is exactly the policy we should pursue with all people everywhere whom we may wish to influence. This cannot be done without a deeper understanding of ourselves, as well as of others, and I hope that these pages may do at least something to further that under-standing, and the consequential ability and power which it may give us.

CHAPTER II

OPENING PHASE OF THE INTERVIEW

EVERY human relationship begins with the interview, and, therefore, it is of the utmost importance that we should not bungle it. By this I do not mean that we should be on our toes, as it were, in a state of anxiety, for that may be the surest way of putting us at a disadvantage, and even perhaps of putting the person interviewed also in a state of anxiety, and ruining the whole thing. Anxiety, at least an undercurrent of it, at interviews is only too frequent. In due course I shall show that such a state of anxiety comes essentially from an unconscious source, and the way of dealing with it is to discover the unconscious source of it. However, at the moment we must content ourselves with the surface level of things. It will not be denied that we should endeavour to make the very best of a first interview, and leave nothing to chance. It may take an infinite amount of time and trouble to put right anything that we have put wrong at the start—indeed, we may never be given the opportunity, for a bad first interview may well make it the last interview. However confident we may feel that we could put everything right given a second chance, the second chance may never come.

To take things in their proper order, one might say that the first contact usually begins *before* the interview. There are the events that led to the interview being sought or arranged. For instance there may have been a recommendation. Much depends upon how such a recommendation was made, with enthusiasm or with reservations, and, above all, by whom it was made, whether or not by one whom the person seeking the interview trusted, respected, or loved. But these are matters over which we, in the role of the interviewer, have no control. Nevertheless, they may have a considerable influence upon the attitude of mind which the person, for instance a patient, brings to the interview. I think physicians are insufficiently aware that most patients coming to a first interview commonly bring with them a considerable amount of distrust of the physician, mixed, of course, with their hopes and fears.

If there is going to be any therapeutic or analytical progress, all these things will eventually, though not immediately, have to be brought to the surface and fully discussed on a conscious level.

Apart from the initiation of the interview, such as by recommendation, there are matters which come within the power of the interviewer to control. The interview has to be sought by letter or by telephone. Our methods of correspondence, promptitude, even our secretary's voice on the telephone, are not without their initial effects. If we ourselves answer the telephone, it is essential to be patient, helpful, and receptive. The slightest sign of any impatience, resistance, or aggressiveness, and we have revealed the cloven hoof of the destructive instinct! Or even undue volubility and we may well have blotted our copy book beyond redemption. The interviewee has made the first move in ringing-up —we do not know with how much temerity. It may require only the slightest rebuff, and he will be put off us completely and for evermore, or, he will arrive with some negative feeling, resistance or hate bottled up within him. All this could have been avoided by a little control, and a few minutes' patience. Besides, the display of emotion or negativism does us no credit. At the best it exposes our childishness, and, perhaps, our unsuitability to be in a position of superiority or trust. The would-be interviewed feels all this, and feels it deeply, even if he suppresses it from his own consciousness. We have started our account with an overdraft!

If we are talking about professional interviews, such as those given by a doctor, psychiatrist, or analyst, it often happens that the patient has been putting off a consultation for a long time, and that he is, at the moment, in an acute state of distress which has, perhaps only temporarily, overthrown his resistances. He needs immediate help. He wants to see us at once. We know that he must be a complete fool to have no idea of the fact that we are fully booked up for the next three weeks, that we have no proper vacancy till then. And what sadistic gratification we may get on informing him of this fact! However, such sadism will rebound to our own disadvantage.

If we are fit to be a practising doctor or analyst, we should be moved primarily by sympathy or empathy for the poor sufferer who needs our help and who is perhaps humiliated to the extent of asking for it. It is no good expecting him to understand our difficulty. A person in an emotional state is like a child or infant: he does not consider how busy mother is—he just cries or screams for her. And if she is a good, kind, loving, sympathetic mother she should go at once. Thus, we should see our urgent, emotionally distressed, or felt-to-be-urgent applicants as soon as they can get to us, or at the very earliest opportunity thereafter, even if we can give them only ten minutes or a quarter of an hour. The proper appointment may be arranged at the same time. We must sacrifice our tea or lunch interval if necessary.

Apart from such cases of urgent emotional distress, which, fortunately, are in the minority, most would-be patients are likely to have their full attention concentrated upon assessing us and our merits to become their helper and saviour. They may have looked us up in the Medical Directory. They will try and form their estimate of us from our address, the district in which we practise, our house, the appearance of the house, our waiting room, perhaps the length of time we keep them waiting. Here I would say that whatever theories one may have of giving a good impression of being busy by keeping people waiting ten minutes or so, we lose more than we gain by such inhuman tactics. If we were in full sympathy with suffering humanity, we would at least endeavour not to keep them waiting at all. A person is commonly in a considerable state of tension before a first interview, before any professional consultation, even with a lawyer. Any professional consultation involves a personal and an intimate relationship, though perhaps none so much so as that with a new doctor or consultant. To some people, especially to anyone suffering from psychoneurosis, the position is emotionally not unlike that of going to meet a prospective suitor. It is natural to start vetting him even before one catches sight of him.

He shows no prospect of being any good to us if he is not tolerant and benevolent. The only clues we have of him are the threads we can grab hold of in advance of the interview. I am reminded of that story of the doctor's baby, left in a pram outside the consulting room. He pointed his finger at every patient that passed and exclaimed: 'Another damned nuisance!' The Doctor's smiling reception a moment later could hardly do more than reveal that there were two sides to his, perhaps understandable, ambivalence!

Eventually the moment arrives, and the patient is ushered into the sanctuary and the presence. Some erstwhile successful political leaders were not indifferent to the psychological effect of their office environment upon callers. One has heard that Mussolini preferred a large marble hall where the caller would have to undergo a long and lonely walk under scrutiny! I believe he preferred also a high desk from which he could look down upon the miserable worm. Incidentally, the psychological effect of our Courts of Law, even Police Courts, is similarly calculated to render helpless and impotent those subjected to their awful influence. In contrast, the doctor's consulting room should, in my opinion, be friendly, cheerful and happy, and calculated to make the pent-up sufferer relax and be at his ease. Our therapeutic objective should not be to 'castrate' him further. He is already ill. He has come to us to be restored, and what does it matter if the scale tilts the other way, and he assumes a critical role of investigation of us and ours. We should be pleased that he is not too ill to be able to do that. There is no need for us to feel that he is getting the upper hand of us. If we need to be on the defensive, we should be analysed before we see patients. I may add that the patient is most likely to get a 'transference' towards us, with its attendant need for our presence and help, if he is sufficiently free from anxiety himself to be able to assess us and our demerits.

If he is well enough, everything about us is going to influence him and unconsciously determine whether he wishes to see us again or not. Our appearance, face and figure, our movements, behaviour, mannerisms, and not only what we say, but the very tone of our voice—all these are going to have more influence upon him, and indirectly upon us, than any of the conscious superficialitites of the interview.

In my young days, when I was under control-analysis, I was temporarily annoyed by a remark of my controlling analyst. I had grumbled about a new patient whom they had given me to treat at the Clinic. I said of him: 'You sent me a patient who is practically incurable, and who is going to stick to me like glue for the next ten years.' The question of my controlling analyst that annoyed me was, 'Did his father have curly hair like yours'!

I mention this to emphasize that fetishistic attachment, nonsensical as it admittedly is, commonly has more influence upon our likes and dislikes, and certainly upon our fallings in love, than would be credited by the unanalysed. However, though we may have little control over it, that is all the more reason why we should appreciate its importance, and understand its overwhelming influence. I shall refer again to this matter in a later and more advanced chapter. There may be a good deal of this type of influence, affecting the patient's reactions, even to such vague attributes as personality.

Undoubtedly, the apparent character, maturity, learning, experience, intelligence, wisdom, and probably above all, *naturalness* of the physician are going to have their effect upon the immediate emotional rapport of the patient. A lot of these attributes are not subject to our will. We cannot help their presence, absence, or degree; but naturalness, at least, it may be possible to acquire, for its prerequisites are a freedom from anxiety, particularly unconscious anxiety in ourselves, and confidence in our knowledge, ability, and competence.

One thing that is going to carry a lot of weight with the patient is, of course, evidence of a genuineness of our interest in him, and the genuineness of our intention to help him, and not to spare ourselves in so doing. Of course this must be coupled with some confidence in our ability to do so. Second only to this, in influencing a patient's positive transference at the first interview, is this thing called personality, and freedom from any vestige of anxiety. These things apply not only in the medical interview, but in any and every walk of life.

Why is it that a particular teacher can take over a new class, even a kindergarten class, and immediately be, without question, supreme master of the situation? The same may apply to taking over control of animals. In an identical situation, another person will flounder or become unnecessarily aggressive, beating everyone up, as it were, with anxiety. The confident and mature adult knows and feels that the others are helpless children. The analyst should know still more deeply that they are chock-full of ridiculous childish anxieties about their infantile, aggressive, and sexual impulses, now fear-repressed; unconsciously terrified lest these horrors are revealed, and no less terrified of knowing the truth about their own unconscious.

This does not mean that one has to assume superiority, or believe that one is a superman—indeed, there is no need to feel oneself in any respect superior or better than others; but a knowledge both of oneself and of them does at least help to make one an adult. The sensing of this personality in the physician or analyst will result in the sensitive patient feeling a certain amount of security in his presence. If the doctor or analyst has succeeded in freeing himself from anxiety, the patient will, provided he knows the doctor is his staunch friend, sooner or later, feel similarly free, secure and relaxed.

This psychological position of the analyst must be a genuine one if it is to produce the desired results, for every patient who is not too ill, will, at a first interview, be observing most acutely, even if subconsciously, every gesture and every change in facial expression. It is impossible to camouflage everything all the time. That is why naturalness pays the best dividends, for at least it rules out the anxiety-provoking element of deceit and suspicion. I would, however, modify this extolling of naturalness by insisting that it does not mean a free expression of one's own thoughts or affective reactions. A physician must be free from the need to reduce his tension in the patient's presence, and must leave that role exclusively to the patient, resigning himself to observation, and, if necessary, encouragement.

Every hesitation which a patient displays is a demonstration of anxiety, analogous to phobic anxiety. The best encouragement will, in the long run, prove to be interpretation of the unconscious sources of his anxiety, but this will, in most cases, prove to be impracticable at a first interview. We will probably have to accept the disadvantages of this superficial defensive situation. We do not yet speak the same language, at least not at a conscious level. We have to accept the conventionally limited vocabulary of consciousness, as though pretending, with the patient, that the greater world below the level of consciousness does not exist.

CHAPTER III

WHAT GOES ON

SOMETIME ago I received a questionnaire from the editor of a popular journal. He had evidently prepared his questions on the basis of those received from readers' letters. I must say that it gave me a shock to realize how incomprehensible any effort to explain the technique of analysis would have been to his readers.

The questionnaire was as follows: 'What actually goes on at analysis? Does the patient sit or lie down? Do you take notes? How long does a session last? How often do you hypnotize the patient? Do you inject willpower? Would alcohol or drugs help the patient to talk his thoughts more easily? How much guidance or advice do you give, for instance, about the rules of living? Does a patient feel different after treatment, and, if so, why and how?'

What was so shocking about these questions was that not one of them betrayed the slightest clue to anything really relevant to analysis, or, as I would here say, to the basic nature of the interview. I found it impossible to answer these questions at their face value without, at the same time, encouraging a totally erroneous conception. I have thought of an analogy to explain what I mean:

Suppose a person had been so isolated from civilization that he had never come across writing and reading—for instance, a savage from the wilds of Africa. When he heard about it for the first time, he might well ask such questions as these: 'Does a person stand up or sit down or lie down to perform this antic with his hand? What instrument does he use to make the marks with? What good are those marks on the paper? Is he asleep or in a dream when he does it? Does anybody feel different after looking at those marks?' If you answer these questions, and a thousand others, do you suppose the questioner would have any better idea of what essentially constitutes the communication of thought through the intermediary of the written word, leave alone any appreciation of the quality of literature or the benefits to be derived from it? It is not unlikely that if you attempt to explain these essential matters to him, he will either not understand you, or he will be incredulous.

In short, neither sitting down nor lying down constitutes psychological analysis any more than it constitutes the communication of thought by writing. The particular posture is assumed only to facilitate the mental and physical operation, and to restrain distracting activities. Similar answers may be given to most of the remaining questions.

Length and frequency of sessions are concessions to reality—the interfering real world outside the mind—and, as such, may be regarded as unfortunate, though necessary, interruptions of the process. This process might *ideally* be continuous, but in this world it is not usually possible to achieve the ideal. For convenience sake, analytical sessions are commonly limited to fifty minutes, but in some cases it is necessary to allow even double that time. Similar things may be said about frequency—the more frequent the sessions the better. If you are pushing a car along, you lose impetus and momentum by taking a rest.

It seems to me that the questioner is unwittingly asking: 'In what ways does reality (actuality) enter into and interfere with analysis?' Actuality is concerned with the so-called real world, and with what is visible on the surface. Analysis is concerned with the invisible processes hidden in the unconscious mind. It is natural, if one has no conception of the existence of these latter, that one should focus one's attention and enquiry upon the surface material, however inconsequential it may be.

I have chosen this excerpt from my experience of writing about analytical material, because analytical interviews underline or bring out, in vivid relief, the neglected or hidden aspects of all interviews. Particularly in the analytical interview, it is not so much what one *does*, nor even what one does *not* do—though that is infinitely more important—it is rather what goes on under the surface, unseen, what goes on under the surface in every interview. The difference between analysis and the interview is that it is the business of analysis, in due course, to bring these unseen things to the surface, to consciousness. They are none the less there in the interview, though we do not then necessarily bring them to the surface. It is the business of this book to tell you something of what they are, and to help you to see that insight into them is the only thing that can influence *appropriately* what we do and do not do at an interview—if we are conducting it. It is these unseen, unspoken events that are the essence of every personal relationship. They are more than unspoken. At almost all interviews we are everlastingly hurrying, as it were, to *deny* them, to deny their existence. We behave as though we were terrified of them.

It is the business of this book to lay these ghosts, to bring as many of the hidden bogies that people can bear to see out into the open, into the light of day. It will be admitted that some of them may reside in the interviewer, even if he is an analyst, as well as in the interviewed. It is the business of analysis to deal with what is called counter transference as well as with transference. The former is due to an unconscious process in the analyst, as the latter is in the patient. It is the business of analysis to deal with counter-transference-resistance, as well as with the patient's resistances. All these things are present, though less obvious, at every interview.

Exceptionally we may meet an 'interviewer' who *enjoys* them, even if he does not know what they are. Such a one is a Maurice Chevalier. He warms the heart. He can fill the Hippodrome with an enchanted audience.

A very introverted and emotionally inhibited patient of mine had reached the stage when he was attributing all his troubles to a lack of emotional freedom which he had experienced with his parents as a boy. He told me that on the long walks which he and his father habitually did together, all their conversation appeared to be limited by a sort of conventionally drawn, invisible, chalk line. It was mutually understood that there were certain subjects— a large variety of subjects—which one did not mention or allude to. They included every subject about which either party might have the slightest feeling, any and every subject that might be accompanied by some emotional tone. Perhaps the nuclear centre of the taboo was sexuality, but, if so, the ramparts and defences around it had been extended so many miles beyond that the chalk line was very near the edge of the playground, leaving a very small and restricted place in which to play, or in which to confine the subjects of one's conversation. It would never have occurred, either to him or to his father, to infringe the rule, even so much as to draw attention to the chalk line. Thereby, they could conduct their mutual contact free from anxiety.

He clearly remembered that on the rare occasions when they

met an acquaintance, and the conversation extended to a group of three, he, on his part, would feel distinctly uneasy. The upsurge of anxiety, he recognized quite clearly, was due to the possibility of this intruder not being adequately acquainted with the rules of the game. Some reference might be made, some subject introduced, which would be an infringement of the convention silently recognized by his father and himself. Hence the uneasiness, and hence the sigh of relief when the stranger departed, and he and his father could continue without any danger of the repressive barrier being breached. It can be imagined what a dreadfully anxious time this man experienced in all his personal contacts until he underwent analysis.

The interview is a sample of personal contact occurring before the parties to it have had their unconscious anxieties assuaged by the reassuring effects of some knowledge of each other. My purpose is to stress that it has an unconscious as well as a conscious aspect. I would go even further than this, and insist that it has also a physiological aspect. Witness, for instance, the all too frequent duodenal ulcer, which occurs in anxiety-ridden or tension-ridden individuals. Such anxieties and tension are provoked or exacerbated especially in connection with the unconscious emotional reactions of personal contacts such as interviews.

Under the broad category of 'unconscious', I would include all the reactions of one person to another which are not conscious and manifest. They are by far the larger and more important category. They are, as it were, the power behind the throne, the really effective determinants of his behaviour, of his decisions. They will affect, for instance, perhaps all unsuspected by him, his determination, whether or not to see you again. They will affect, as it were, his 'expression' beneath the mask, perhaps visible sooner or later through the mask. They will affect not only the battening of his eye-lids, and the intensity of his heart beat, but even the chemical constitution of his blood . . . and of his gastric juices, (witness, for instance, diabetes, duodenal ulcer, functional colitis, heart disorders, rheumatism and the whole conglomeration of psychosomatic disorders).

In most 'How to . . .' expositions the whole phenomenon of the unconscious, mental, physiological, and organic, is neglected. 'How to Make Friends . . .' and so on! ('How to Add Two

Cubits to your Stature!' Was not that debunked two thousand years ago?) This is what makes such books, however popular, so useless. We might pause for a moment to ask why they are so popular. Perhaps the answer is that everybody is seeking for an answer to his anxiety problem. The place he never dreams of looking for it is below the surface of consciousness, the other side of the chalk line which my patient and his father drew. Such books are based on the utterly false premise that our conscious ego rules us and our work. This is an illusion. The contrary is the truth. Unfortunately, I can talk and write only to your ego. Whether any change will penetrate below that level by virtue of reading this book will depend upon the strength of your resistances, and upon how successful I may be in wooing you from their influence.

I would not say that the conscious aspect of an interview, or of anything else, is of *no* importance. The lipstick a lady puts on is not of no importance, nor the way we do our hair, or clothe ourselves, nor the mask we wear to keep ourselves and others from being frightened by the fears or lustful animals beneath it. But must we all be taken in by masks all the time?

Believe me, what lies beneath the mask is infinitely more interesting, if you will take courage from me or from any other analyst, and not be too frightened to look at it. Analysis shows us that it is better that way because practically all our ills are the result of things operating beneath the mask, and catching us unawares—because we were too frightened to open our eyes and see what was there. Actually it is only nature—God and devil— and all that proceeds out of the mind of man. Even the mask bears some of the imprint of its unconscious origin if we have eyes to see.

All this is by way of explaining that when I analyse the 'interview', it will be more its unconscious than its conscious aspects that will concern me. Pretence we have in abundance, and will continue to have. Can I give you a glimpse of something that lies beneath the pretence? Can anything short of analysis enable one to open one's eyes, and see what is there? It did so happen in the case of Freud, and I have met other unanalysed persons whose experience and intelligence led them to considerable insight without analysis, but this is far from true of the majority. Most of us spend our lives being pushed about by forces of which we have no cognisance.

To illustrate the difference between the conscious and un-conscious aspects of the interview, I will relate the following analytical excerpt. Once upon a time there came to consult me a great financier, who was the proprietor and director of a dozen companies. He said to me: 'Although I employ hundreds of thousands of people, if I have to interview the lowest labourer amongst them, I *feel* like a little boy in the presence of a grown-up man. What makes it worse, what makes it more of a strain, is that I have to *pretend*, and keep on pretending, that I am perfectly at ease. I have, by hook or by crook, to maintain his illusion that I feel like a great employer. Can you cure this outsize inferiority feeling, Doctor?'

This great man had, as it were, risen from the ranks. His father had been a village fruiterer. The fright of his life had been his father's bankruptcy, and the family's semi-starvation. That was when my patient was barely fifteen years of age. His whole life, including his business and economic success, was anxiety-driven. (Here, again, it would be misleading to suggest that the actual conscious event of the family bankruptcy and starvation were the fundamental cause. They were a rational and visibly precipitating stimulus.) The real cause lay in his unconscious anxiety-complex, stimulated, or I should say re-stimulated, so powerfully at fifteen years of age.

What was wrong with this man was, of course, that he felt an 'id' or instinct-level immaturity. He felt that inside himself he was not really grown up. How can emotions develop and mature normally if one has grown up in a sort of panic? Something in him sensed or felt an immaturity . . . and most acutely when he had to act the superman, to maintain an inflated prestige.

At this interview with his employee much was going on at both a conscious and an unconscious level. The two levels were not in harmony with each other. On the conscious plane he was the superman; on the unconscious plane he was still a frightened little boy in the presence of a grown man. This grown man was un-consciously associated with his father-image and made terrifying by his own unconscious guilt, and by a projection of the repressed, aggressive, hating and destructive impulses of early life. Techni-cally, of course, it would be no good telling him this at a first interview. He would have to find it out for himself by degrees, as I am hoping the reader may, in part, through a progressive study of this book.

At the interview, or at any other personal contact, one may be unduly sensitive, or unduly insensitive. I remember, as an undergraduate, sitting in the amphitheatre of the Hospital Out-Patient Department. The surgeon was in an elevated position, seated at a high desk. On a low chair beside him, near his feet, there sat a humble patient. The surgeon was holding a tape measure which had just been used. Out of contempt for some student's answer to his question, he flung this measure into the air, and, more or less unseen by him, it fell across the head and face of the patient seated beneath, and dangled over one eye of the awe-struck man, who remained sitting there motionless and terrified. There was plenty of emotion in the air. I was not the only spectator who felt unexpressed anger far exceeding that demonstrated by the surgeon. Recognizing the emotional content of personal relationships, conscious or unconscious, does not mean necessarily that we draw attention to them.

To end on a more pleasant note; looking from my window I see a young couple, two adolescents, boy and girl, who have been knocking up at the tennis net. They are now in conversation across it. Perhaps they are talking of stroke-production, or the weather, or what not. An interview is going on. Its conscious content can hardly matter very much, but if one analyses their movements and their inhibitions, including a certain tense embarrassment, nods and smiles, a jerk of the head, and a swish of the racquet behind the back, one may easily guess that a lot more is probably going on at an unconscious level, even at physiological and glandular levels. Otherwise, how does anything important biological, especially reproductive, happen on this earth?

What does it matter if a first interview, or an acquaintanceship between two people, begins with *defence* predominating, defence often covered with a camouflage of a positive nature. The libido is merely feeling its way, through anxiety, towards some gratifying expression of itself.

Can we maintain the fiction that the important reactions at an interview, or in any personal contact, are those which appear on the surface?

CHAPTER IV

THE PURPOSE OF THE INTERVIEW
AVOWED AND UNAVOWED

THE conducting of an interview naturally depends upon the conscious or actual purpose for which it is taking place. Most of us try to maintain the fiction that this is all there is to it. Usually we get away with this illusion more or less successfully. Sometimes the actual purpose of the meeting makes this easy. There may be no need even to look at the salesman when, for instance, buying a packet of tea. We can treat the whole transaction as automatic, as though we were putting our money in a machine, and pulling a lever, ruling out practically all possibilities of unconscious or emotional reaction. However, I think it may be admitted that even for such mundane things as purchases, especially if they be of a more personal nature, psychological factors are tacitly recognized by the profession of salesmanship.

The physician, the psychiatrist, and even the analyst, would be well advised to take note of the principal slogan of salesmanship, namely that 'the customer is always right'. It is a tacit recognition of the fact that the average customer will, one, forego even the wanted article if he has to face a negative emotional situation to get it, and, two, that if the emotional situation is pleasing and gratifying to him, he is likely to purchase articles which he would not otherwise purchase. We have joked amongst ourselves about some enormous Car Servicing and Repair Works, where the owner-driver is met, not only by a workman or mechanic who knows the job, but also by a gentleman representative of the firm who conspicuously knows nothing technical, but whose function is clearly that of dealing with the customer's emotions! Amongst one's friends he is humorously called 'the flannel man'.

All this is by way of suggesting that, whatever the overt or avowed *purpose* of an interview may be, every interview has its psychological element. I am tempted to suggest that in most interviews the psychological element so outweighs other factors in its importance or in its potential effects, that one might be justified in saying that, irrespective of purpose, every interview is a psychological one. Even in trade or salesmanship, if we forget or disregard this fact, we may get our packet of tea thrown back at us.

If this were a more advanced chapter, I would be inclined to go further, and to suggest that the difference between the actual purpose of the interview and the hidden psychological goings-on is not really so different as it would seem. Both have at least one thing in common, and that is the relief of dissatisfaction, tension or frustration, and the acquiring of some modicum of satisfaction. We are all busy relieving ourselves of discomforts, and trying to acquire comforts, whether this operation is going on in relation to actuality, material, chemical and physical, or whether it is taking place in phantasy, phantasy stimulated by personal contact with one another.

In short, even the avowed purpose of an interview has its direct and indirect aim in satisfaction, *a psychological quality*, and in some interviews the actual placebo or toy for this satisfaction becomes secondary to the emotional phantasy connected with the personal relationship. It is on this account that the general principles developed in connection with medical and analytical interviews are applicable to almost all interviews. No matter what the avowed purpose of the interview, it often so happens that our need to relieve ourselves of tension, and to use the other person—the person whom we are interviewing—as a therapist for this purpose, overrides the reality or actual purpose for which the interview was arranged. It often happens that we are in such great need to unburden ourselves of our tensions that, to a greater or lesser degree, the other person is used as a therapist irrespective of his unsuitability for the role; and, I would emphasize, irrespective of the probable fact that *he* requires a therapist or analyst upon whom to relieve *his* tensions.

Very often the better business man is the one whose need for emotional relief in these, often unconscious, ways is successfully subordinated to the conscious purpose of the transaction which he is pursuing. If he can implement this by encouraging the other party to use him as a confidant or therapist, he will probably gain all the advantages (other than the immediate emotional ones) from the interview. Thus, to be a good business man often means to be a good therapist, however unconsciously.

The corollary to this is the truth that a person who is in urgent need all the time of relieving his emotional tensions, from whatever source, and who is, in consequence, apt to pick upon any and every opportunity of personal contact to use the other person, however unsuitable, for the role of 'therapist', is himself unfit to be a therapist or analyst. So far as psychological help to his patients is concerned, he may be unfit to be a doctor or general practitioner, though I qualify this by saying that the insensitive man who has unduly repressed all his emotional life, and put on too hard an exterior, may be even less suitable.

If, for the sake of clarity in discussing the purpose of an interview, we reject such displacements as sale of goods, achieving of appointments, assignments and so on, and confine ourselves to the basic emotional reciprocity, we may say that it all depends upon whether the interview is designed for our emotional benefit or for that of the other party. It all depends upon whether we desire or require the interview for our personal emotional relief or for that of the other, whether we intend to help him or to help ourselves. We should be clear in our own mind as to which it is. Otherwise, there is the risk of confusion of purpose and the possibility of mutual irritation or exasperation (e.g. a row), instead of emotional relief to one party or the other.

To simplify the discussion, I have elected first to describe the technique of an interview at which the other party is to receive mental benefit. Now, I do not wish to encourage or to nurse the illusion that we can, as a matter of practical politics, for ever be dispensing emotional-mental benefit to others, without receiving or requiring anything in return. We are not saviours of mankind; and, if we would dole out benefit without return, we shall, whether we know it or not, be surreptitiously taking in benefit—emotional benefit as a rule—be it only that of building up a Christ-complex for ourselves.

I happen to know a doctor, a specialist, who has become so inflated by the worship of his women patients that, when he deigns to talk to one, he lifts his chin a little higher with every priceless remark! No doubt there are some who would prefer to do without the benefits he bestows, but his academic success is such that he

B

still has plenty of patients, despite his God-complex. Maybe a high proportion are taken-in by it. But let us not forget to be charitable —it may be, of course, that the poor man is self-conscious or shy.

However, the purpose of this reference is to emphasize that this man has certainly never been psycho-analysed. It would be impossible for any analysed person to be like that. He would have become too conscious of too many truths about himself. The exception to this statement would be: unless he had a tic, the source of which was so sub-mental that it had eluded treatment! The analysed person does not 'help', or annoy, people by exhibiting a 'superiority complex', or an overt reaction to inferiority feelings.

Well, assuming that our interview is designed for the therapeutic benefit of the *other* party, it is necessary, not only to avoid Christ-complexes, but also to avoid negative reactions on our part, however controlled and repressed. To avoid these it is necessary that we ourselves should be receiving equivalent benefit. If we are not going to receive this on an emotional plane, we must arrange that our satisfaction should, nevertheless, be there, usually on a conscious, material, or economic plane. It should be avowed (not denied), admitted and conscious to both parties to the agreement. In other words, it is necessary for the therapist, as well as for the person receiving psychological benefit from the therapy, that the former should receive a fee in exchange.

What I have wished to stress is that, if the therapist's need for emotional relief overbalances his need for satisfaction in the fee, the tables are liable to be turned, and the patient will be made into the therapist. He will almost certainly, like such a therapist himself, be quite unfit for the role.

I once knew a doctor who essayed analytical work without having previously subjected himself to a course of analysis. An interesting situation arose. A patient who had been sent to him, complained that, when he described one of his dreams, this analyst spent the rest of the session telling the patient one of his, the analyst's, dreams! Subsequently this patient told his doctor that he did not pay fees to listen to the dreams of any consultant.

Of course, this may not have been so ridiculous as it sounds. It may be that the patient had told a dream and stopped, and this analyst felt he could encourage the man, and give him more confidence, by showing that he could dream equally foolishly. It may be that the patient was the hostile, complaining sort, looking for an opportunity to pick holes in one who presumed to set himself up as teacher, mentor or analyst.

I mention this analyst as a hint that we are all probably doing something of the same sort at our interviews, and though it may not be as inappropriate as this, the difference is more of degree than of kind. In other words, our would-be therapy is, to some extent all along the line in various ways, vitiated by our unanalysed need to use the other person as a therapist, and to burden him with our undischarged tensions and complexes.

On the other hand, I have known patients complain that we do *not* do enough of this: 'How can I go on telling you my troubles, Doctor, when you do not tell me yours?' But this is nothing to the complainings that would ensue if we did! This brings me to the subject of the next chapter.

CHAPTER V

THE INTERVIEWER AND THE INTERVIEWED

THE late Dr. Rickman used to say that until now, psycho-analysis had pretty well confined itself to what he called the One-Person Psychology. I was a little surprised to hear this, as, in my experience, stress has always been laid upon the psychology of the therapist, together with the emotional interactions between him and the patient. Indeed, as far back as 1928, Dr. Glover emphasized that the difficulties of psycho-analytic technique are conveniently resolved into two groups—those incident to the patient, and those incident to the analyst. Of these he stressed that those incident to the analyst were the more important.

In the recent issue of the 'Annual Survey of Psycho-analysis', the statement is made: 'The most important field for investigation of this coming theory (namely, the theory of the relationship of one person to another) is the analyst's relation to his patient, and its libidinal implications'. Thus, I have good authority for considering the interview firstly from the point of view of the *interviewer* and his psychology.

Whatever the nature of the interview, analytical or ordinary, it is essential that the interviewer should be free from any overweening need to relieve tension, anxiety, or to unburden his complexes. Otherwise, like the analyst I mentioned in the previous chapter, he will be liable to reverse the roles, or at least to make the interview one of reciprocal emotional sharing. Admittedly each party to such an interview may receive a modicum of relief or satisfaction, and, at the same time, a lesser or greater amount of frustration or vexation. This is the nature of most of our personal contacts. The characteristic of the social interview in contradistinction to the therapeutic or analytical interview or session is that in the social interview each party uses the other for his relief, irrespective of whether such relief is bringing satisfaction or increased tension to the recipient. In any case both participants will be subject to their own unanalysed resistances, taboos, and limitations.

Thus, the emotional level is liable to be of a superficial nature, so far as its conscious mental elements are concerned. The degree of satisfaction will be limited in proportion to the personality limitations of the individuals participating, each being subconsciously concerned to avoid the arousing of anxiety in himself if not in the other.

The picture reminds one of the instance I mentioned, of the boy and his father whose mutual exchanges were conventionally restricted, as it were by unspoken agreement, so as not to infringe the chalk line, that is to say, not to run any risk of emotional provocation. To the analyst it is a sad fact that most of us live our lives separated from an emotional vortex by a flimsy chalk line, or more often by a wall which we are ever endeavouring to reinforce in relation to the increases of pressure on the other side of it.

A certain amount of anxiety gets through and is experienced by the ego when pressure threatens—which is practically all the time. But the sad part of it is that we are denied mental participation in the rich and dynamic life which goes on on the other side. Our inhibitations are our 'safeguards'. Analysis reveals that there is not the slightest need to be terrified of all these terrors. If they are wild animals they are found to be only infantile ones, and, with adequate recognition and exposure, they can be sufficiently well handled by the adult ego.

The purpose of recording all this is to emphasize that the good interviewer, like the good analyst, should not only be in control of his emotional tensions and complexes, but should ideally have few unsolved problems and few overweening complexes. To be a good analyst, one must go further, and have a very sound conscious knowledge of all the important tendencies in one's unconscious mind. Otherwise, when the interviewed, or the patient, displays emotions—particularly emotions directed towards oneself—one's own unanalysed complexes will be aroused, and one will be liable to enter the emotional dog-fight of ordinary passionate relationships, instead of remaining outside it, as an analyst must, and having control and power over it.

I am reminded of a patient from abroad who had been treated by an unorthodox lay analyst. Not only had this analyst been inadequately analysed, but his own personal emotional life had not been satisfactorily adjusted. In consequence he had reacted to the patient's positive transference feelings, and their libidinal accompaniments. He was in similar need himself. It was an inadequate excuse that the patient was a rich young widow, too neurotically ill to be likely to achieve any marital adjustment. It was an inadequate excuse on account of the man's 'professional' role regarding her. Increasing emotional disturbance led her to seek my advice. At the very first session she brought me a dream in which she and her late therapist were reclining in a car that was travelling at speed, firstly over undulating ground, and finally over very bumpy ground. In the end it started to career down hill. She then noticed that there was nobody at the steering wheel; there was nobody in control. She was terrified, and awoke screaming.

Perhaps it does not require an analytical training to interpret this dream. To have a sense of security in life, and adequate freedom from anxiety, is a prerequisite of the peace of mind which is necessary for enjoyment. Libidinal freedom does not relieve tension unless it is accompanied by the security which confidence and control alone can bring. This patient was too neurotically infantile to feel confidence in her own controlling abilities. She was in need of an analyst as a child is in need of a parent. But the analyst's function should be primarily that of reducing her anxiety, not increasing it, and, through the transference, interpreting its sources, until her own ego is in a position to take charge.

To be competent to achieve this, the analyst (or interviewer) must be free both from unconscious conflicts himself, and from emotional frustration with its attendant need for emotional relief. Similarly, the analyst must be sufficiently free from complexes in himself not to react to a patient's negative transference, abuse, and hostility. He must recognize that expressions of hate, however vituperative, are to be encouraged to the nth degree. Repressed hate and aggression are the very stuff of which morbid and psychotic symptoms are made. It is because they have been repressed and damned up in the unconscious that the patient is ill. Expression of them, particularly with the analyst as object, is a most important step to freedom through therapy.

Of course, the analyst must analyse, that is to say interpret, them and reveal the source from which they spring; but he need not hurry to do this, provided the patient is continuing to give adequate vent to them. Interpretation should be if anything for the purpose of encouraging their expression rather than because we are disliking the attack for personal or unanalysed reasons. Any sign of resentment on the part of the analyst at such attacks will ruin his treatment; even undue silence may do this.

There are some patients, who at certain stages of their analysis are constantly trying to provoke the analyst into a quarrel or argument. If he allows his emotions to be aroused, so that he falls for this, he is degrading his "therapy" to the level of the ordinary sort of dog-fight, and the treatment will surely fail, and fail when success was most promising. I know that it is said that negative transference, in contradistinction to positive, should immediately be analysed, but I am sure that the main purpose of interpretation should always be that of removing resistances, and enabling free association of thought, the basis of the analytical movement, to continue freely. This rule takes precedence over all others; and some patients, most patients, require to express an enormous run of hostility *unchecked* by the need of the analyst to fend it off by interpretation. In short, the analyst should be so well analysed himself that he has no difficulty in seeing, in the patient's abuse of him, that patient's infantile conflict with his parents. He should not be in *too* great a hurry for the patient to see it.

Perhaps this is the essential difference between the analysed and the unanalysed, namely, that the analysed person, at least if he is acting in the role of analyst, should be able to endure the patient's hostility without reacting to it, without having his own hostility aroused. If he cannot do this, he requires more analysis himself, or if he cannot do it in any special instance, he will have to send that particular patient to another analyst.

I am admitting that it is natural for any person to react to hostility with hostile feelings, and this is one of the two reasons why the analytical interview is so far superior to ordinary personal relationships in its therapeutic effects. The other reason is interpretation of, instead of reaction to, positive libidinal affects. These are the two strongly emotional sides of the transference: love and hate. In analysis we are not afraid of either of them; we are not taken-in by either of them; we do not react to either of them. We interpret any resistance to their expression when their expression tends to be resisted; and, when the time is ripe to interpret them, we do so. They are always the projected expression of an intra-psychic conflict between the patient's id and super-ego (with the ego taking alternating sides); and this intrapsychic conflict was originally a conflict between infant and parent (or parent surrogate).

It may be added here, in parenthesis, that the State—which should be the greatest and kindest parent figure—might well learn something from these analytical revelations, instead of behaving towards its children like the primitive, barbarous parent of the Stone Age! (I do not mean by this that the State, any more than the parent, should allow aggressive children to injure it).

The purpose of this exposition of the analyst's attitude, and of his emotional and ego relationship to his patient, is to suggest that the interviewer could not do better than model his 'technique' upon this rather ideal example. If he is sufficiently free from tensions, complexes, and the need to relieve his own emotions, he will find that, in so far as he successfully operates this technique, to that degree will he obtain the transference of the interviewed. Not only will he be benefiting the interviewed emotionally and mentally (ego), but the interviewed will feel gratitude towards him, and a tendency to put himself in his hands, to lean on him. This will do no harm to either party. If the interviewer has not only these capabilities, but is himself benevolently disposed, both participants may have everything to gain from such a conduction of an interview or personal relationship. The questions that one must leave unanswered are, how far an unanalysed person may succeed along these lines, and whether any person can be adequate to such a task unless he knows that he is on duty, receiving recompense for the sacrifice of so much of his potential emotional gratification.

In short, the interviewer has to make his choice between selfish emotional gratification and the satisfaction of sympathetic and benevolent feelings with real personality-potency and power. Furthermore, it may not be entirely a matter of choice, as the emotional forces within him may be too compulsive to permit him a great deal of choice in the matter.

PARTS I AND II: THEORY

PART TWO

THE INTERVIEWER

TYPES OF INTERVIEW
ACCORDING TO PURPOSE

CHAPTER VI

THE HOSPITAL INTERVIEW

WHAT a fascinating subject is medicine! In the last quarter of a century such advances have been made in the chemical, physical, and bacteriological aspects of medicine, that our power over a variety of diseases has increased beyond recognition. The discovery of the sulphanilamides[1], and even more especially of penicillin and the antibiotics, have revolutionized treatment. I imagine that all wise people anticipated that research in physics (even apart from nuclear-fission), chemistry and biochemistry, would, in due course, revolutionize medicine and beyond-medicine.

Nevertheless, contrary to popular belief, medicine still contains many more unsolved mysteries than triumphant solutions. There is, for instance, that enormous list of psychosomatic diseases, diseases which have now been almost generally admitted to have a psychogenic aetiology, or at least to be accompanied by, if not preceded by, outstandingly important psychological factors. Perhaps the most generally accepted of these is peptic ulcer. In my student days it would have been considered irrelevant, if not crazy, to give phenobarbitone to the sufferer, but now I believe it is almost routine.

Cardiovascular diseases (from essential hypertension [high blood pressure] to angina, and even heart failure), and rheumatism, with rheumatoid arthritis, are the commonest psychosomatic illnesses, each accounting for (according to Dunbar) twelve per cent of human disability and invalidism. Nervous and mental illnesses are said to account for eighteen per cent. But the list of psychosomatic (i.e. psychogenic) organic diseases includes also: allergies, such as hay fever, asthma, and (?) the common cold; respiratory disorders; endocrine disorders, such as thyrotoxicosis and diabetes; nearly all skin diseases (certainly all the common ones); vasomotor and blood diseases; some epilepsies; migraine; effort-intolerance, and accidents.

Perhaps it is not necessary to stress the magnitude of medi-

[1] Sulphonamides is a more generally used term than sulphanilamides nowadays.

cine's unsolved problems. Its relevance to what I am going to say is this: I do not believe that in hospital and in general medical practice any advance in psychological medicine has been made comparable to that achieved in physical, chemical, and bio-chemical medicine.

When I was a student at St. Thomas's Hospital, nearly half a century ago, there prevailed at that time in all teaching hospitals, a rigid convention that the people who applied for treatment, whether out-patients or in-patients, were simply 'cases', samples of various recognized diseases. It would have been almost a breach of etiquette, as it were, to have got to know any one of them personally, as an individual. I imagine that fellow students, as well as doctors, would have looked at one askance, wondering what on earth one might be up to in attempting any such approach. Besides, how on earth would anyone have the time for such a thing, such an irrelevant form of investigation? It may be that some general practitioner (poor thing!) could not entirely escape it, but in hospital it would have been little short of an outrage. Our time was fully occupied in the physical and pathological examinations of the various diseases presented, as it were, by these specimens or carriers of them. So far as any psychology was concerned, they might have been a lot of test tubes, carrying their germs, or what-not, in culture.

The Form of case paper which recorded the medical clerk's or student's Interview with the patient more or less emphasized this attitude. After name and address and date, it started with something like this: 'The patient is a married woman of 52, complaining of . . .', and then there were about a line or two in which to record what she complained of. Subsequently there were a few lines for her family history, and then for her past history—each, of course, strictly with reference to the complaint. And, then, perhaps, a page on which to record the history of her present illness.

The student would take these things down as quickly and briefly as he could, hardly looking at the patient, except in abstract, while he did so; for he was hurrying to get into his stride when he came to what might be regarded as the proper business of the case-record, namely, the physical inspection, a detailed physical examination, concluding with laboratory tests,

X-rays, and what-not. This important document, also, had its precise formal pattern, beginning with a few lines devoted to the general appearance of the case, followed by an inspection of the mouth, tongue, and throat. It then proceeded to details of the examination of the various organic systems in rotation— cardiovascular system, lungs, abdomen, central nervous system, muscle, skin, concentrating naturally upon any particular part that appeared to have special reference to the complaint. Laboratory and other tests would subsequently be recorded.

The mind was almost, though not entirely, left out of consideration. There was plenty of excuse for this; to begin with, one had quite enough to do attending to what were regarded as the relevant physical matters; but I am sure that the real reason for leaving out the mind was because it is, or might become, dangerous ground. This statement is not so absurd as it may seem at first sight. For one thing, it would surely be natural for any person in contact with another, first of all to engage himself in studying the other person's mind, however superficially. It is much more natural, and, indeed, much less of an effort, to do this, than to start strapping blood-pressure apparatus on to the other person's arm, or to dig out stethoscopes and listen to his heart and lungs, and all that sort of thing.

But if it is natural to listen to a person whom one is there to study, and to concern oneself with his complainings, his character, nature, and interests, why is this hurriedly side-stepped in favour of an impersonal physical investigation? I think the answer is that it is tacitly recognized that if once we got the patient loosened up, and freely expressing himself, it might be almost impossible to stop him. There would be no end to it, and he might be an impossible pest, voluble, and perhaps a little undisciplined, interfering with one's calm and peace of mind, and handicapping one's time and one's freedom in physical examination. Therefore, the doctors in hospital, particularly the students and the young doctors, find it safer to keep the patient's personality at bay. They give him no alternative but to keep that side of himself bottled up. They do not want his emotions; they want to be left in peace to pursue their physical, chemical, and bacteriological investigation.

What I would here like to stress is that the very existence of this natural phenomenological liability (i.e. the psychological outpouring on the part of the patient) indicates, to my mind, that it is what the sufferer, the patient, really needs. But, never mind, he is accustomed to bottling it up; probably even his general practitioner does not want it, has not the time for it, and he could hardly expect the scientific investigators in the hospital would want to be bothered with it. They do not.

However, there is another aspect of this matter (dichotomy between mental-emotional and physical investigations) which is possibly the most relevant. It is this. So long as a physical examination is performed by a stranger, an official in an official position, it has a better chance of being and remaining an impersonal, unemotional matter. You are being examined by an 'instrument', as it were, something which, from an emotional point of view, you might regard as that elaborate conglomeration of valves and wires, which the physicists flatter themselves by calling 'a mechanical mind'. The physical intimacy is less likely to disturb you emotionally than a similar performance by a fellow human being, who is felt to have a personal relationship to you, however recent and superficial.

And from the other point of view, if the hospital examiner thinks of you only as 'specimen number twenty-three', he will avoid any *emotional* interest in you, and your blessed body. He will be interested solely in its germs! *In short, the interview and contact designed by hospital and medical-physical examination is characterized by safeguards or resistances against the arousing of any personal feelings or emotional reactions. If it is an interview, it is an interview with the characteristic of the avoidance of mental intimacy, even at the expense of the avoidance of mental knowledge.*

In spite of all this, I have seen a patient, a young woman, too emotionally inhibited and nervous to have made any successful alloerotic or love contacts in her life, who may be said to have been suffering from a 'hospital-perversion'. Her sexual life, apart from autoerotic activities, was confined to the 'perversion' of getting herself medically examined on various ingenuous pretexts by unknown doctors, such as those she would encounter in the out-patient department of a hospital. The thrills she experienced at these 'impersonal' physical contacts can be compared only to those which the normal person would feel in ordinary sexual love relationships. Of course, it was due to her morbid anxiety that she could only enjoy such matters provided they were under the effective cloak of a non-sexual situation.

But apart from such exceptional abnormalities, perhaps a large proportion of more normal people would not be entirely cold to physical-medical investigations *if* it were the practice for the examining doctor to precede his physical investigation by getting them to unburden themselves mentally to him beforehand. The mental unburdening would, sooner or later, be liable to lead to a transference, or emotional tendency, towards the person who received it, and if, thereupon, that person proceeded to any physical approach, however medically authentic, a considerable proportion of fairly normal persons would be liable to react emotionally, as though a lover were touching them, however one-sided the reactions were likely to be.

An excerpt from my own experience may serve to underline this theory. I had had a number of sessions with a middle-aged married lady, who complained, amongst other things, that she had always suffered from total and absolute sexual frigidity. At this session she had grumbled chiefly about rheumatic pains in her left shoulder. They were so severe that they extended right down to her finger tips, affected the left side of her chest, and caused her to worry lest her heart were involved. When the session was over, and she stood up to go, I was curious to know whether she really had any osteo-arthritic changes in that shoulder joint. Being aware of the sort of material which I have been here recording, I hesitated for a few moments, but then took the risk, hoping that a transference to me was not yet sufficiently established for there to be any harm in such a cursory physical approach. I put my left hand on her shoulder, outside all her clothes, as she stood facing me, took her elbow in my right hand, and did the familiar passive rotary movement to diagnose crepitations in her shoulder joint. She left the room in silence.

At the next session she could talk of nothing else but this physical contact with me. She said: 'When you touched my shoulder, I felt myself go rigid all over. I tried not to show it in my face, but I made all my feelings go completely dead. I was absolutely anaesthetic everywhere. You could have stuck a pin in me, or even a knife, and I would have felt nothing'.

Incidentally, this has an interesting bearing upon the psycho-pathology of her frigidity, particularly when she attempted to answer my questions. I said, 'Why did all this happen, why did you do this?' I put the question: 'Was it necessary?'

Her reply was: 'It was an automatic reaction on my part, and the reason for it, I am quite sure, is that, if I had not taken those precautions, *the opposite* would have happened. I might have lost control.' Later, she went on to say: 'I would have got an orgasm when you touched me, and would have felt such a fool that I would never have been able to come here again.'

The relationship between psychological transference, which comes about through the process of unburdening one's thoughts and feelings mentally, and emotional response to any physical contact, is thus made vividly clear by such an intensified instance as this.

In the hospital interview, all that doctors and patients are doing, in view of the physical-examination-programme, is just what this patient did automatically when I touched her shoulder. The essential difference is that they, doctors and patients alike, are exerting this automatic, or almost instinctual, defensive process well in advance, at the outer perimeter of the emotional or orgasm-giving citadel, the citadel which has to be defended against intrusions that the ego has not arranged or accepted. This form of the conventionally accepted guardedness is thus a characteristic of the medical as distinct from the psychological interview and investigation.

CHAPTER VII

THE DOCTOR'S INTERVIEW

THE general practitioner or 'family' doctor is in the invidious position of having to be part psychologist and part 'hospital' or organic-disease-doctor. He is subject to all the difficulties and dangers which this double role incurs, and, therefore, there is every excuse for him, if taking his cue, as it were, from his hospital training, he adopts a defensive attitude, and blocks all the emotional overtures, which some of his patients so persistently hurl at him. In due course he may get a bit softened up, but his chief stand-by or safeguard can still be his great busyness and pressure of work.

I have had experience of this role myself, and know it sufficiently well and intimately to be able to give some first-hand information. Almost all the patients who come to the general practitioner desire and require psychological help. This does not only apply to the large majority, the patients with 'nothing (organic) the matter with them', but it applies also quite definitely to those who are physically or organically ill. Apart from the likelihood of their organic illness being of the psychosomatic or psychogenic variety—even if it is one of those that are conceivably not so—the patient is suffering; and every person who is suffering. from whatever cause, mental or physcial, needs psychological help and relief. The child who falls and cuts its knee does not merely require the plaster and bandage. He also, perhaps primarily, requires comfort and relief of his psychological distress. Practically all adults, whatever they are suffering from, if they go to the doctor, are basically children, and require psychological comfort as well as physical attention. They need a kind and able 'parent', as well as a scientific instrument. Nevertheless, the important psychological factors are commonly, as it were by tacit mutual agreement, hidden beneath the mask of the physical need.

To quote from Henderson and Gillespie's *Text-Book of Psychiatry*: "No new psychopathological discoveries are to be expected in this field (the field of psychosomatic medicine); but light may be thrown on the relationship of mental to physical illness, and on the possibility of psychogenic functional reversible physical changes becoming permanent, irreversible or even structural'.

These words need careful study by those who are not familiar with this sort of phraseology, for they refer to a familiar succession of events—one, a mental or emotional change, such as we experience in anger or fear, leading to, two, physiological or functional changes in the body, including physical and chemical changes. (Such changes, I may say, accompany every emotion and every shade of emotion; no emotion is possible without its having repercussions of a physical and chemical nature upon the body and its functions.) Three, the changes produced by an emotion, can, if repeated strongly and frequently enough, become permanent, so that they become irreversible or unable-to-be-undone; and, four, such changes can produce even alterations in structure of certain organs or parts of the body. This last condition would correspond to organic disease—the chain of events having started on a mental or emotional plane.

Henderson and Gillespie go on to say: 'What these studies so far emphasize is the need for treatment purposes of taking account of the whole man, i.e. the need for a psychobiological viewpoint in clinical medicine as well as in psychiatry.' What Ryle says of the visceral neuroses is true of disease in general: 'The story of the "visceral neuroses"—heartburn, spasmodic dysphagia (difficulty in swallowing), globus (hysterical lump in the throat), colonic neuroses, vasovagal neuroses, cardiac neuroses (paroxysmal tachycardia and vaso-vagal attacks)—is a story of men and women, of personalities and temperaments, of hereditary habits and evironments.'

Thus, even the most orthodox and accredited exponents of medicine and psychiatry are nowadays pointing to the fact that illness, functional illness, and even organic illness, cannot be separated—as hospital practice used to incline us to think—from the 'story of men and women, of personalities and temperaments, of hereditary habits and environments.'

This is, *par excellence*, the province of the general practitioner, of the family doctor, of the man who knows the persons, the personalities, the families (and environments), as well as the particular ills from which they suffer, who has interviews and personal contacts with them all.

In addition to his smattering of organic disease cases, the practitioner has a large number of patients whose sufferings are still principally mental or psychoneurotic. These, too, have their secondary or associated organic changes. Although there is no psychological experience, even a passing emotion, that does not have some physicochemical accompaniment, the tacit agreement between patient and doctor is that the latter will concentrate upon the physical side—even if it is not large enough for the methods of clinical, or even of laboratory, medicine to find anything abnormal.

A third variety of patients that present themselves are those who have failed to adapt themselves to life. It may be that the ordinary habits and activities demanded by life are a bit too much for them. In psychological practice one sees more marked instances of this sort of thing. My own theory is that these are cases of mental defect in the direction of schizophrenia, though without being diagnosable as such.

For instance, I saw recently an adult patient who could not cope with the ordinary routine activities of life. She told me that when she was a school-girl things were already almost too much for her to manage, though she struggled on and kept her place amongst the others as best she could. Tragedy arose when she reached puberty, for, thereupon, the extra bit of adjustment necessary to cope with her menses—the matter of sanitary towels, what to do about them, and, particularly, how to dispose of them (apparently without discovery)—was the last straw. She could not cope with any more, and she then had her first real nervous breakdown.

A fourth group of patients that come to the practitioner are, of course, the admittedly mental ones—cases of severe psychoneuroses and psychoses. Nowadays a large proportion of these seem to be the depressives—only less hopeless, from his point of view, than the aggressive psychopaths, or impossible characterological cases. The point is that all these people, from first to last, suffer both in body and soul.

The practitioner cannot avoid some mental involvement with each and all of them, and he cannot maintain the emotionally disinterested attitude, or the element of aloofness, which used to be, and perhaps still is, the defence, not only of the hospital doctor, but also of the classical psycho-analyst. Moreover, unlike the psycho-analyst, he cannot escape what the patient regards as his essential duty of physical examination. Certainly his position is an extremely difficult one. He should be free from anxieties, if not a bit of an adventurer at heart, in order to stand up to it. I think he ought not to be left to learn *all* his psychology exclusively in the hard school of experience. A great American doctor, now deceased, one who had never been psycho-analysed, wrote: 'Two persons who speak to each other are in a social relation (in the wider sense of the word, *including the erotic relation*)'.

Can the physician maintain the parent role sufficiently in spite of his psychological relationship to his patients, and in spite of having to couple it with physical examination, perhaps frequent physical examination? How does he achieve this marvellous feat without the safeguards of either the hospital physician on the one hand, or the aloofness of the psycho-analyst on the other?

Perhaps it all goes to show that if we must draw lines, it does not really matter very much where we draw them. Perhaps all our defensive systems are really more reactions to morbid anxiety than due to their having any real justification in the nature of things. The important matter is simply that the ego should remain in charge of affairs, whether they may be the emotional affairs of the instincts within, or the reality affairs of the world without.

But general practice certainly has its compensations as well as its difficulties. Of all varieties of professional work, it is, I think, the one that puts the practitioner in the closest, most complete and most satisfying relationship to the largest number of people of the greatest variety. When I say satisfying relationship, perhaps I should add, particularly if one likes the role of the important benefactor and respected father-figure.

I well remember the many occasions, when having knocked at a front door, I have been confronted by a hostile, suspicious, and scowling housewife. Possibly she thought I was some tax man or rent collector! I have merely said the magic word 'Doctor', and watched her expression change to one of benevolent and respectful affability: 'Come in, Doctor; this way please. It's our John, we have been so worried about him'. What could be an easier introduction to an interview? What other profession could expect such treatment so consistently?

I have known many practitioners, particularly in country districts, who found their profession so satisfying to every part of their personality and nature, that they were usually reluctant to tear themselves away from it to do anything else. A wife in a country district complained to me of her doctor husband: 'He won't join me in the lounge after his evening surgery until late at night. Even when he can't spend any more time with the patients, the last one having gone, he is so fond of the blessed place that he potters about amongst the *bottles* for hours'!

Unless one *enjoys* being father to a large, troublesome, but usually grateful, family, numbering potentially some five thousand souls, it would probably be better to adopt some less emotionally absorbing profession.

But now to focus our attention more precisely upon the doctor's interview with his patient. In most ordinary or industrial practices the doctor's chief reality concern is time. He has so much to attend to, and so many people to attend to, that life would be quite impracticable if he were to relax and indulge himself in the sort of psychological investigations and considerations which are the stock-in-trade of the analyst. For the practitioner, brevity is an essential commodity. On this account he is usually very wide awake to the first remark, the first sentence, which a patient pronounces, whether in his surgery or at a visit. He knows, from experience as well as from habit, that it is most important that nothing arises to defer or becloud the patient's first statement.

It facilitates his time-saving object to receive the patient politely, to sit him down, and himself to say nothing, or next to nothing, until the patient has spoken. This, of course, is the ideal behaviour on the part of any interviewer. One should be completely receptive, and say only the minimum that is necessary to get the patient, or the interviewed, to take the lead. The interviewer's function is merely to put him sufficiently at his ease, so that he will not have any inhibitions, and will express himself as soon as possible. The doctor who receives his patient with a lot of volubility is probably overdoing the encouragement technique—perhaps on account of his own anxiety. In most cases we have only to allow the appropriate situation, and the patient will speak.

I used to try and make a practice of writing down the first

words he said. Occasionally a patient, usually a woman, would start with: 'Doctor, I am afraid I have got cancer.' This would be enough in practically all cases to establish the diagnosis: 'Anxiety state'! Of course, one would 'have to let her talk on for a while; naturally with due regard for other patients in the waiting-room! But in view of the time factor, one would take the first opportunity of satisfying her expectation, and examine the alleged cancerous region. Never once have I been introduced to real cancer in these terms. Reassurance might then be complete enough for the time being, but, of course, this was the sort of patient that one could depend upon turning up in the very near future, and again and again. She would always be needing reassurance about something or other, if not physical examination.

The reference to general practice or family doctor is of interest in reminding us that there can be no rule-of-thumb for the interview. Experience, and his natural or acquired personality and tact, tell the doctor that every single person he interviews requires a technique appropriate to that particular person. In short, on these cursory lines of interview, it would not be incorrect to say that there are as many techniques as there are persons to be interviewed. Our intelligence and experience and instinct alone can teach us what is most appropriate. What suits one may be grossly inappropriate for another.

This reminds me of an 'interview' with the big fat pleasant housewife who, years previously, had been seeing me with a fresh complaint almost daily. The family had moved out of London, and, after a considerable interval, she reappeared, looking as usual the picture of health. This time she had a scrap of paper listing a hundred and one complaints. (I believe Charcot used to speak of *'la maladie à la petite pièce du papier'*!) I was very busy, and my waiting-room was full. I let her get through her list at the expense of ten minutes of precious time. I then rose to my feet. She automatically rose also, and said, with some display of excitement, 'But, Doctor, tell me what is the matter with me?' I turned her towards the door, and smacked her great flank, remarking, 'You are a big, fat *goose*, and that is *ALL* that is the matter with you!' She went out roaring with laughter. I am not suggesting that this variety of interview would suit every general practitioner, and certainly not every patient!

Each person requires his own appropriate technique, but in these interviews, as in all others, the practitioner should be master of the situation, particularly master of himself and his own emotions, never lose his temper on any account with anybody, be always polite, courteous, and show that he has a genuine regard for the personality of the individual consulting him, take seriously everything the patient says, including even his wildest theories, never laugh at him or make fun (unless he knows his ground very thoroughly indeed) and, in general, act up to the role assigned to him, of sympathetic, competent and reliable parent.

At the same time, he should not himself be taken-in by this role, and even if his patients endow him with magical powers, he will be gravely disillusioned if he begins to believe in them himself.

In my opinion he will do best, and enjoy his profession most, if he is free from inhibiting anxiety, particularly inhibitions or repressions of natural emotional response to the patient he is interviewing. It is sufficient if he has control, and if his own sexual life is satisfactorily adjusted.

If only the general practitioner had sufficient time at his disposal, and sufficient instruction and encouragement from the right sources, he is the man who might, above all others, above the hospital official on the one hand, and the psychiatrist or analyst on the other hand, be in the best position to investigate the enormous new and developing field in medicine, namely that of psychosomatic illness, an appreciation of which, in my opinion, will become the next great advance in medicine.

CHAPTER VIII

THE PSYCHIATRIC INTERVIEW

CAN we learn anything from the psychiatric interview, a very specialized affair indeed, that can be applicable to interviews in general? I think we can learn a great deal, both of a positive and of a negative nature, things to follow, things to bear in mind, and on the other hand, things to avoid.

Firstly, it should be said that the psychiatric interview has naturally to be modified, sometimes beyond all recognition, according to the severity of the mental illness of the person being interviewed. For instance, we could hardly have an interview in any ordinary sense with a stuporous mute, or even for that matter with an acutely maniacal patient. But, for descriptive purposes, one naturally has in mind the more usual type of case that could be led to answer one's questions.

We are assuming that the object of the psychiatric interview is primarily, one, diagnostic—to diagnose the type of illness; and, two, to decide what would be the appropriate procedure, such as where and how to place the patient for treatment. This latter naturally depends upon the degree of severity of the illness, the prospects of amelioration, etc. Also it is usually the interviewer's business to prepare a detailed case paper, embracing all the relevant facts and information.

But, perhaps the most outstanding difference between the psychiatric interview and all other interviews is the fact that in the case of the majority of psychotics there is a relative or absolute *absence* of the matter which I regard as essential to all other types of interview and personal contacts—namely, a *rapport*, a lively or intense emotional relationship (largely unconscious) between the interviewed and the interviewer.

A characteristic of psychotic cases is that they are mentally and emotionally more or less withdrawn into themselves, withdrawn from reality and from emotional reciprocity with those in touch with them. In short, they have largely severed their contacts with everything outside themselves, and withdrawn into their own inner world. It is often very difficult, and in some cases impossible, to enter it with them or to draw them into ours. The barrier may be impenetrable, but not necessarily entirely so.

However, at the interview the interviewer has to perform the definite tasks to which I have referred, and he has to exercise a very special technique in order to overcome the obstacles which the unco-operative patient may present. In most cases he will have to have an interview with the nearest available relative, perhaps with several relatives or friends, in order to get a description of the patient's conduct, and, perhaps, a history of the illness since its onset. Indeed, he may have to compile almost the entire case-paper from information received from people other than the patient. The formula for such a case-paper, whether obtained from the patient or from others, is in outline very much the same as that used for psychoneurotic, or indeed for any other medical case-paper, only perhaps rather more detailed and compendious.

For instance, one will need a *family history* with separate treatment of the father and mother, including not only recognizable mental difficulties, but also such things as alcoholism, eccentricities, and peculiarities of every kind. This must be extended to each parent's relatives, even for two or three generations. Then there is the matter of brothers and sisters. A record must be made of each, particularly, of course, with reference to mental peculiarities in every blood relation.

We next come to the *personal history* beginning before birth. The question of the mother's health during conception, prematurity, difficulties of labour, weight at birth, breast-feeding, age at weaning, type of babyhood, infancy, particularly with reference to infantile neuroses, such as night terrors, bed wetting, tantrums, backwardness and other peculiarities.

Presently we come to school life. Here we want particulars under the headings of class performance, physical prowess (games, etc.), and social adaptability. Puberty must be carefully gone into, and adolescence. Naturally any previous nervous or mental disturbance or abnormality must be carefully recorded. It is a curious fact that in spite of such detailed case-takings, many psychiatrists find themselves apt to forget, perhaps until the last minute, the frequently all-important subject of sexual development. It is astonishing how often, coming back to remedy this omission, one discovers, particularly in the psychoneuroses, that the essence of the aetiology lay specifically in this department. How universally this is a part of even normal cultural development may be judged from the fact that it is *usual* to have some symptom in this connection. It commonly takes the form of excessive reaction-formations, neurotic defences, prejudices, biases and phobias. However normal *behaviour* may be, these reaction-formations create morbid scotomata (blind spots) in the mind, and make it impossible for many so-called normal people to consider this particular subject objectively.

Eventually one comes to the history of the *present illness,* an important object here being to try to discover any and every factor which may have contributed to the precipitation of the illness. These should be recorded with dates and age of the patient at the time. We want to know at how early an age certain interferences with psychological development took place, and what they were. We want to know the patient's reaction to changes of his circumstances throughout his life, and, of course, especially just prior to his breakdown or breakdowns. We want to form an estimate of his disposition, temperament, and character, and the way he has reacted to any special stresses in his life. If the first interview is properly handled, from this point of view, we may get more factual information on the spot than we are likely to get at subsequent contacts.

Physiological functions and events should also be inquired into, such as menstrual irregularities, illnesses and operations, sexual habits, including perversions, love attachments, any addiction to alcohol or drugs. Our mind will naturally be concentrated upon an investigation of the first deviation from the normal. The question of sleep and sleeplessness is of outstanding importance. We should not hesitate to ask if there have been any suicidal tendencies.

In our personal interview with the patient, while we are assessing his faculties, mental and emotional, his degree of guilt-feeling or apathy, memory, and so on, we need not generally hesitate to ask him such startling questions as whether he has been hearing voices or whether people have been behaving strangely towards him.

I remember once seeing a young man in my waiting-room, because I was unable, owing to my time-table, to give him a proper appointment. His mother had brought him round because he had been brooding in a way that worried her, and behaving peculiarly. For instance, he had been sitting on the stairs as though rapt in thought, sometimes far into the night. His manner was a bit strange, but when I asked him what was the matter, he would only insist that there was absolutely nothing the matter with *him*. Yet it was obvious that there was. Suddenly I turned to him, and asked, 'Do you hear voices?' He immediately jumped to life, nodded vigorously, and replied, 'Yes.' Then, with enthusiasm: 'It is the neighbours. They keep talking about me. I can hear them through the walls when I sit on the stairs.' That was all I needed to know, for I was not proposing to take the case. I telephoned a colleague who was in charge of a private mental hospital, and everything was fixed up immediately.

The point about psychiatric case-taking is this: Generally speaking, these patients are so withdrawn that it is inadvisable, and usually unsuccessful, to pester them with details of the questionnaire, answers to which we so urgently require. If we try that method on them, we are likely to arouse their resistance, so that they become less and less co-operative. A very special technique is required, and we need a fair amount of time for it. I should say that all psychological interviews should be unhurried. The technique is to let them talk if they are inclined to talk, and if not, simply to try to get them talking, not in answer to questions, the answers of which *we* want to know, but rather to get them to talk just what they are feeling and thinking, or day-dreaming about. Then we must settle down and listen. We may learn a lot more this way than we would learn by any amount of questioning.

Having learnt all that we think we can learn by simply listening, or by listening and encouraging them to continue, we then tactfully introduce a little enquiry, as the opportunity arises from the subject matter about which they are speaking. For instance, if the patient has been talking about his sister, when he has finished, we may ask if he has any other sisters, or brothers, and so lead him on to give us the family history. Admittedly, it may sometimes be better to get all this from somebody else, and confine our examination of the patient himself to encouraging an exhaustive recital of his own mental pre-occupations, particularly if they include delusions, hallucinations, and psychogenic sensations and symptoms.

Many psychiatrists like to make as scientific an assessment as possible of the patient's intellectual ability, memory, both recent and remote, orientation in time and place, what is called apperceptive ability, i.e. ability to assimilate and to comprehend, insight and judgment, adaptability, or, more commonly, lack of it. Of course, all this is subject to the patient being well enough to endure it, and well enough not to be unduly irritated or provoked by it.

For practical purposes the patient's general activity and behaviour are of special importance. In institutions patients are segregated, that is to say, appointed a particular ward, in relation to their *behaviour*, not in relation to their diagnosis.

It goes without saying that a thorough physical examination should be done in every mental case, perhaps with special concentration on the central nervous system. Analysts who are in the habit of confining their activities to the purely psychological aspects of illnesses may be excused if they prefer to delegate physical examination to a general physician or neurologist.

What we can learn from psychiatric casetaking is, not only the helpfulness and satisfactoriness of having a systematic case-paper of a person, but, most particularly, the principle for application to interviews in general, of refraining from putting the interviewed through a teasing and irritating cross-examination in order to gain our end.

The technique of psychiatric case-taking which we should apply to interviews in general is that of allowing the interviewed to express himself unchecked, and to subordinate our need for information to the principle of giving him freedom to express himself. The technique is to try to glean the answers we want from what he says unquestioned, and if that is not enough, to guide him or lead him ever so gently and most tactfully into giving us some of the information which we require. It is usually better to sacrifice the gratification of our curiosity, rather than to arouse annoyance and resistance in the course of gaining it. Perhaps we can gain it some other way, at some other time, or from some other person. An exception to this principle, if it is an exception, is one which is, perhaps, applicable only to psychotic patients, and it consists in not hesitating to ask direct questions about such things as hallucinations and delusions. Far from such questions being offensive and insulting to the psychotic, he often grabs hold of them like a hungry man, and is delighted to give us all the information we require with an eagerness and volubility which were entirely lacking in regard to all the factual matters of our case-paper in which he is relatively uninterested.

CHAPTER IX

THE THERAPEUTIC INTERVIEW

N o w the psychiatric interview, as described, is a piece of work which is conducted almost exclusively by the interviewer's ego. He uses his intuitive tact, of course, but perhaps only to the degree of checking himself from bursting in and interrupting the patient's needed self-expression. The patient is one whose ego is deficient, or temporarily so, and there must be at least some ego about, so the interviewer has to supply a double share of it. I am inclined to feel that in the therapeutic interview almost the opposite is the case. I should say that by 'therapeutic interview' I mean an interview designed simply and solely to relieve the interviewed of his distresses and tensions there and then, at that particular interview. I may say that it has also a remote valuation. Most people, particularly ill people, are activated, whether they know it or not, by what we call the pleasure-principle (even if his 'pleasure', at the moment, is merely a reduction of his anxiety), and you would hardly expect a person to come rushing along, pleasure driven, to tell his vexatious cross-examiner more relevant facts about family history, seeking a second and third interview for such a purpose. On the other hand, if the person interviewed has, as it were, enjoyed himself by getting a great deal of trouble and tension off his chest, unchecked and sympathetically received, it is more likely that he will have some desire (pleasure-principle) to return to the sympathetic recipient, in order to pour out a bit more.

I once knew a colleague who possessed, in unusual abundance, some rather dumb sympathetic aura. Indeed, I have sometimes, rather uncharitably, suspected that his mind was so absorbed on the sympathetic and emotional level, that there was very little room left for ego activity. His method of conducting an interview, or rather the tangible results that accrued from the interviews he conducted, had nothing to recommend him to the approval of a medical superintendent or psychiatric teacher. Indeed, it might almost be said that he did not bother to *conduct* anything. He must have had some genius for making his patients comfortable and relaxed, but beyond this I imagine there was no conducting. As far as I can make out, he asked not a single question, though he did have sufficient reality sense to observe the clock, and that, considering all the other attributes of his interview, seems rather incongruous. A patient would leave him after an hour's talk, without, believe it or not, his knowing even the patient's name and address. He did not bother to interrupt her to ask such a question. It seemed to him, as, possibly, to her, irrelevant.

Once when he was discussing a patient, something arose, and I said to him, with surprise: 'But you have learnt nothing of her family history, or anything else about her.' He replied, very aptly, 'Do you hasten to learn this when introduced to a new acquaintance?' And he added, confidently, 'The point is, the patient will come back . . . to-morrow.' And she did.

I can still remember my astonishment in my young days when a doctor told me the patient I had interviewed had decided to go to *another* analyst. I hurriedly unearthed my case notes, wondering where I had gone wrong. There was a complete case history, one of the best and most compendious I had ever taken. It consisted of nearly twenty pages of hurried scribble, embracing, in proper sequence and outline, every conceivable aspect of the case, in my opinion, the model of a psychiatric interview. And after all that, the patient had decided to go to another analyst! Perhaps, that was why! It occurred to me that I must have given her a most gruelling hour and a half in order to elicit all that information, in such detailed completeness. What made it even more humiliating was the fact that she was an exceptionally brilliant and highly educated woman, actually with a double-first honours degree. Probably that was why I made the mistake of assuming that she could not only take the gruelling I must have given her, but that she would be favourably impressed by the thoroughness of it. Anyway, that was the last I saw of her. I have reason to reflect that my unsystematic friend, relaxing in a chair across the room, and possibly thinking his own thoughts, perhaps getting no information whatsoever, confining his activities to sympathetic noises, might well have scored success where I had failed. This is why I suggest that the therapeutic interview may well be the antithesis of the psychiatric one. Let us take this lesson to heart. There is a lot to be learnt from it.

Now the point about therapy is that it is very difficult, if not impossible, for the unanalysed and ego-orientated interviewer to appreciate its principles adequately. One sees patients who obviously have a lot to get off their chest. As soon as the interviewer says the word, 'go', so to speak, they are off. They talk and talk. Only too often their talk appears to have no chronological sequence, and sometimes it is irritatingly inconsequential, without rhyme or reason, and it is difficult to see that it is leading us anywhere. In these circumstances what we should note is the amount of affect or emotion which accompanies their ramblings. So long as they are getting some feelings off their chest, they are probably gaining something from the interview, although we ourselves may feel we are getting nothing satisfactory.

From a therapeutic point of view it is probably best just to let them go on and on uninterrupted, even if, however hard we listen, we can glean nothing very much. We may console ourselves by thinking that at least they are abreacting. Abreaction—another word for relief of pent-up emotions, often without apparent context—is temporarily beneficial, temporarily therapeutic. They will probably go out feeling better, and attribute the betterment to us or to our skill, although the only skill we have exercised is that of not interrupting, and not asking questions or leading the session in a direction which would not give them this desired emotional relief. Further than this, one can say that if one does interrupt and ask questions, one will thereby be damning up the flow of their discharge, and causing them to feel frustration, discomfort and anxiety associated with us, instead of good feelings. This will operate in the direction of losing the patient instead of keeping him, however reasonable or even necessary our questions may seem to be to us. In stopping his natural outlet and trying to get the information we want, we are, *from an emotional point of view*, seeking *our* satisfaction or gratification, and preventing the patient from having his. He will not like us for it, and may never come again.

I could go further than this, and say that in all such cases as the one I have alluded to, which may comprise the majority of neurotics, there is *no other course* than to let them come and talk, and continue to come and talk, until the thing begins to peter out on its own. Then, indeed, our knowledge, insight and technique will be required, if only to interpret why the flow has ceased. But what I cannot emphasize too strongly with reference to a first interview, and every interview, is that *no other treatment* is going to satisfy this type of patient, or begin to satisfy him, until he has been given the opportunity to get off his chest everything that will come out spontaneously, together with its attendant emotions. Anything more or less than this will be worse than valueless; it will be frustrating.

After all, we may say that this type of patient is doing spontaneous free association of thought, even without having been told what it is, or that it is the basic rule of analysis. He is doing it spontaneously, and what more could any analyst desire? Such a patient may, with more or less help, go through all the familiar early stages of analysis. He has already got some preliminary transference to us, and, while we do not interrupt him, it is increasing.

Of course, sooner or later, a crisis is inevitable. It may be that he will suddenly tell us, perhaps after only a few such interviews, that he has finished all he has to say, that there is nothing more to say; and he assumes his treatment is at an end. This is where the analyst comes in, and interprets the resistance, which may, by now, be a transference resistance. The fact is that he has more or less exhausted his pre-conscious material and found himself at the first barrier between conscious and unconscious levels of his mind. Unless this crisis is properly handled, with insight as well as with sympathy, the interview or interviews may end.

However, in the meantime, such a patient will have improved to some extent. Probably his symptoms are better, though he has not really embarked upon analysis, for repressed hostilities are still repressed, and the important sources of his neurosis are still untouched. Nevertheless, in view of his spontaneous improvement, however superficial, we may be justified in calling such an interview, or series of interviews, therapeutic. More than this, as I have said, they may prove to be the beginning of real analysis, and by real analysis, I mean transference analysis, an analysis in which the emotional life appears to be concentrated in the present situation between patient and analyst. This is a stage of analysis in which the patient is, unknowingly, reliving his early life, in which the basis of his neurosis was laid down.

c

However difficult it may be to get a patient to pass from this spontaneous opening stage to the stage of analysis proper, the point here is that unless one allows his nature to take its course in this way, unless one allows him to unburden his mind as nature prompts him to do, one will not only be interrupting the therapeutic process of the immediate interview, but probably checking the analytical process altogether, and destroying any chance, however flimsy, of his passing on to the more permanent and lasting therapeutic process.

Of course, not every therapeutic interview develops quite so easily as the type I have described. There are many patients, including very neurotic ones, who at a first interview will show *resistance* to surrendering themselves to this unburdening. They may be very hesitant, or even silent, though obviously pent-up and distressed. They are, perhaps visibly, in the throes of a conflict. They have come to us to tell us everything, and something is stopping them.

Their conflict, like all conflicts, consists of two parts. The first is a deep-seated desire to get relief. If this were not present somewhere in their psyche they would not have come at all. The second is an inhibition, resistance, or hesitation, to letting this unburdening tendency express itself. Therefore, the resisting or repressing forces in them will have to be more or less dealt with or removed before the unburdening tendency can reveal itself, and get under way. The analyst is accustomed to such situations at many of his analytical sessions, if not at all of them. It may be that experience alone can tell him the appropriate technique to use at that moment in any particular case.

The inhibiting tendencies are obviously anxiety or associated with anxiety. Reassurance is not the usual technique at deeper stages of analysis, but at a first interview it may often be the best we can manage. At any rate, it may be natural to try it first, and, of course, it will be given in a form appropriate to the particular person and occasion. Many patients, perhaps the majority, are naturally a bit reticent or inhibited when they first enter the room. Here the chief reassuring technique of the analyst is for him to be sympathetic, and obviously free from anxiety himself. When they have been motioned to a chair, and asked to make themselves comfortable, if they are still not very forthcoming, it is often a good plan to ask a few emotionally irrelevant or mundane questions, such as the patient's name and address, and to take the opportunity to get a few ordinary particulars while we are, as it were, marking time. These particulars may not necessarily be so irrelevant, though, as factual matters, the patient is likely to take them as a necessary routine, which does not cast aspersions on his inhibited or emotional condition. The particulars I refer to are such things as age, married or single, how long married, number and ages of children, occupation of husband, and so forth.

Finally, if the patient has not taken matters into her own hands, it is usual to ask the question: 'What do you complain of?' or 'Could you tell me now what brings you to see me?' Very often such ordinary behaviour is enough to give the patient time and courage to come out of her shell. As she comes forward, we become silent and sympathetically receptive, speaking only when the patient is silent, and speaking chiefly in order to get her going again, although we may, at the same time, be taking the opportunity of compiling the case-sheet information which we desire.

This sort of interview with a new patient is also therapeutic, but probably only in proportion to the amount of relevant emotionally charged material which she releases from inhibition during it. Thus, the essence of the therapeutic interview is the relief which it gives to the interviewed, particularly if it is impracticable for her to continue the process in the form of regular psychotherapy or analysis.

Patients who do continue pass from what might be called a series of interviews through an increasing facility of self-expression—expression of previously repressed feelings, ideas and memories—to what becomes analysis proper. In some respects this is very like a continuous therapeutic interview.

In analysis proper there should be none of the customary reticences, tactfulness or inhibitions on the part of the patient. Absolute freedom of expression of emotions and ideas, however personal, is the objective. Recently a patient at this deeper stage of therapy said to me—or, rather, yelled at me: 'Shut up! You have tried too many interpretations, and not allowed me enough free-wheeling. I have my strong emotions (much has already been released by analysis), and if I can't let them out, by God! I'm b——, because I was stopped in childhood. I have my strong emotions, and an equally strong ego that stops me letting them out adequately. Don't *you* stop me with your interpretations. If I were to prescribe my own treatment I'd say you should have left me with more free-wheeling, and less of your stuff. I'm not kicking against anything. I'm expressing something that *has* to come out—*for my health.*'

This is an actual verbatim excerpt from an advanced analytical session. I should add that it was shouted at me with a volume of sound that made the rafters ring. Anyone who knew the facts of this man's analysis would say that I had been too incredibly passive and quiet throughout. Enough 'row' emanated from him to occupy the whole of the air. Nevertheless, he is shouting down even *absent* interpretations. He is prescribing his own treatment: 'I'm expressing something that *has* to come out—*for my health.*' He might have added: 'Anything that stops me, even temporarily (such as interpretations) is not therapeutic. It dams me up, and makes me ill, that's what happened in my childhood; and that is why I am ill. I will not allow it to happen again, here. And I will not allow you to make it happen.'

Perhaps this case also illustrates the analytical dictum that analysis *proper* begins only with the *expression* of the *negative* transference. After all, it was frustration and dammed-up aggression, hate or the death instinct, that caused the illness. Expression and relief alone can cure. Therapy aims at facilitating this expression and relief, and subsequent understanding.

The Therapeutic interview is one which encourages unchecked self-expression, particularly the expression of what was previously repressed, dammed-up inside, and wrecking its destructive powers, all unseen, within the unconscious level of the psyche, inaccessible to ego modification.

But this may be passing beyond the scope of a first interview. Perhaps we shall hear more of it at a later stage of this book.

CHAPTER X

A SIMPLE EXAMPLE OF A
THERAPEUTIC INTERVIEW

AN example of a therapeutic interview, now obsolete enough to be recorded, was that of a woman of twenty-eight, now deceased. She arrived in a highly emotional state, but, unlike the popular conception of the average hysteric, under a visibly intense control. The interview had been arranged through her family doctor as an emergency that very day.

Before she would tell me anything, she got me to swear to secrecy, particularly must I promise that, under no circumstances, would I give her doctor—the one who had sent her to me—the slightest clue about what was worrying her. I could see immediately that it was imperative that I acceded to every request of hers to the full. That is to say without quibble, doubt or hesitation.

Gradually the 'terrible' story unfolded. She was now a respectable and well-respected married woman with two children, one of school age. She said: 'It's my father, Doctor. It is so terrible, I don't know how I could have had the courage to come here to tell you. Nobody else must ever know about it. I still see my father. He comes round to me and my husband, has a meal with us, talks and plays with the children, just as though nothing had ever happened. All my friends, too . . . I cannot imagine what it would be like if anyone knew.

'Oh, well, I suppose I shall have to tell you, as that is what I have come for. It was when I was a little girl about nine years of age. My brother six years older. . . . By the way, Doctor, I live rather a long way from London, and I am very tied up with my house-work and looking after the children, so I don't think I would be able to come to you again for any treatment. Besides, my husband could not afford it. Under these circumstances, is there any point in my telling you my secret?'

Distrust and doubt were closing the heart that fane would open. Obviously a little encouragement had to be given. She continued:

'My brother, six years older, had become sexually interested in me. I think it had been going on for some months, perhaps a year. It had developed. One day my father came into the bedroom, and caught him at it.'

'At what?'

'Well, I suppose he was having intercourse with me. My father sent him packing off, and then he, my father, locked the door, and proceeded to do it himself. Really, Doctor, I don't think it had much meaning for me at that time; I was a bit surprised, but that was all, I think. Anyway, I felt that I must not say a word of it to anybody. My family was in very humble circumstances. My father was on night work all the time, and my mother was out at work every day. This practice of my father's continued very frequently for some years. When I was about thirteen or fourteen my periods started, and it was at that time that I took a dislike to it. I told my father so, and he immediately stopped. And we went on with our lives just as though the thing had never happened.

'And so it has been all these years . . . just as though the thing had never happened; although, of course, it has always been in the back of my mind somewhere. Why have I come to see you at this stage, when I am twenty-eight? No, it isn't that my father has turned up again recently, no more than he has always done. We have always seen him at intervals, once a week or so. Of course my husband suspects nothing. Nobody has any idea. No, it's just that something—I don't know what it is—has recently caused me to be worried. Lately my mind has kept going back to this matter and worrying about it, more than it has ever done before in my life, and that tendency seems to have been growing, not getting less. It has led to this feeling, that I must consult somebody who knows about these things, who could understand.'

Some therapeutic value in such an interview may be obvious on the surface, but when the story and a brief discussion of it were over, I felt it relevant, particularly in view of the mystery as to why the old skeleton should have come out of the cupboard and the worry increased so markedly of late, to ask the patient a few questions about her current sexual life. It then transpired that since the birth of her second child, now four years old, her husband had taken to the regular practice of a contraceptive measure, which previously he had only used occasionally. This was, of course, the familiar process of *coitus interruptus*, or withdrawal. Most psychiatrists will recognize the relevance of this clinical material, perhaps the commonest physical cause of anxiety states in married women.

She told me that, since the practice was instituted some four years ago, her capacity for sexual satisfaction had more or less steadily decreased. Eventually she had gone through a stage of disinterest, mounting to frigidity. More recently she had been developing a positive antipathy towards everything sexual. Worse than this, she admitted that, for the first time in her married life, she had experienced some antipathy towards the husband, to whom she had previously been devoted. The sequel to all this was the worry, to my mind possibly heralding an outcrop of neurotic symptoms of the anxiety neurosis variety.

A matter the importance of which could hardly be assessed at a single interview, but which is of some passing psychological interest, is her subsequent association of thought. At this point she told me that she now remembered that during those years of incest, her father similarly regularly practised withdrawal. Thus, there may well have been a psychological, as well as a physical, factor involved in the precipitation of her neurosis, by the recent and cumulative-in-its-effects practice of *coitus interruptus*. However, I am inclined to think that the physical factor alone, in keeping with one's professional experience, might well have been sufficient aetiologically as a precipitating factor. She was, of course, told that this practise must cease, and healthier contraceptive measures substituted. I understand that she was not troubled any more, but many years later she was unfortunately killed in an accident.

The point about this excerpt at this stage is that, apart from the clinical findings of *coitus interruptus*, it serves to illustrate, in the psychological sphere alone, the obvious fact that at least a modicum of mental relief of tension can be achieved in one interview, by a person being uninterruptedly permitted to discharge the pent-up worry, or the particular form of it, which appears to have been gnawing at the mind.

The conducting of such an interview is, of course, simplicity itself. The main technique is that of refraining from introducing oneself unnecessarily, and facilitating the process of the interviewed expressing everything that she wished to express in every detail. Finally, letting her depart feeling that she has been perfectly understood, and that everything is now going to be all right.

The principle of the therapeutic interview is obviously applicable to many aspects of life's activities besides that of a professional consultation. We all rush to friends to unburden ourselves of our immediate current worries. Probably a good deal of our social conversations are, as it were, prophylactic or preventative interviews of this nature. The compulsion to do these things is perhaps greater, more of an 'addiction', than is generally recognized; housewives gossiping to each other over the garden fence, inviting one's friends for a meal, and even the crowded bar at the Local . . . what is going on in all these places? Perhaps it could all be regarded as attempts to get relief by talking, healing interviews in miniature, with their accompanying transferences and counter transferences.

The difference between these and the professionally conducted therapeutic interview is surely that we doctors, professing therapy and accepting a fee for it, should have a better, a deeper, a more conscious knowledge of the patient's psychological forces involved and, *without being pretentious*, know how best to manipulate them for the benefit of the distressed individual who has come to consult us. But I hope to return to this subject, and to give some indication of its deeper aspects and implications, in the course of the following chapters.

CHAPTER XI

THE ANALYTICAL INTERVIEW

THE analytical interview is a mixture of the psychiatric and the therapeutic, with something of its own in addition. This something-of-its-own is that the analyst has to have his eye on the development of the transference. He cannot afford to disregard entirely the idea that he will mirror the patient's transference better the less he has obscured it by an intrusion of his own personality. Therefore, an analyst tends to be much quieter and more unobtrusive at an interview than does the average doctor or psychiatrist.

His endeavour is to get the patient to tell his own story in his own way. Unfortunately, this interview is often, at the same time, a consultation, from which the doctor who sent the patient expects to receive the ordinary case-sheet type of factual information, together with diagnosis, prognosis, and recommendation. Also, the analyst, being a bit of a psychiatrist himself, usually would himself like to have the information as a guide or outline in future dealings with the case, especially if the patient should embark upon an analysis.

Success in these 'materialistic' particulars, however desirable, must, in my opinion, at the analytical interview *be subordinated to the technique of transference development*. In other words, the patient's 'satisfaction' must be placed first, and the analyst and doctor's satisfaction must dance attendance upon it. I previously emphasized this (in chapter nine) by saying that one can get a very good case paper and lose the patient.

We have all been the victims of interviews, of personal relationships, and of social frustrations and annoyances because we were not given the opportunity to express ourselves fully, or because we were contradicted or discredited in some way. Nothing of this sort must happen to a prospective patient who comes to us for an analytical interview. It would be a very bad beginning for transference, for analysis. It would be our own fault if it were the end of the matter.

The way I compromise between the principle of getting the

patient to talk freely without interruption, and the case-sheet ambition, is by asking my case-sheet questions either before the patient has settled down to talk, or when there is a silence to be filled. I ask them almost, as it were, in lieu of the ordinary social gambits—name, address, occupation, how long have you been at that work, and so on.

But, even then, the sooner they can be put aside, however incomplete, in favour of an uninterrupted study of the patient, the sooner the patient can be successfully encouraged to come out of his shell, the sooner will the real emotional matter of the interview, and of the subsequent analysis, get under way. In short, it will be seen that the difficulty of an analytical interview is just this compromise between what I am inclined to call a natural 'id' method of approach, which may elicit little or no factual information an approach comparable to that of the therapeutic interview, and on the other hand, what I call the 'ego' approach, comparable to the psychiatric case-paper compilation.

The question is what proportionate admixture of the two should there be in the compromise. I have little doubt that when I started on analytical work my answer would have been on the side of the ego approach, but the longer I have been at this work, the more prepared have I become to sacrifice any or all of this in favour of the patient's expressing himself in a manner which *he* finds satisfactory. Why should he be made to go to the trouble of fitting everything into our silly pigeon holes. His need is more urgent, more emotionally to the point, and, therefore, probably more relevant, no matter how much it frustrates our desire for case-sheet clarity.

I referred previously to the instance of a colleague whose patients came back though he did not even bother to take their name and address; I still feel that this is going a little too far, but I think what has inclined me more and more to the view that the ego approach should be subordinated, and even, at times, discarded, in favour of the patient's unimpeded emotional expression is my actual clinical experience. The patient who has really become free, who has entered fully into an uninhibited transference stage, does not hesitate to shout one down, or even to tell one to shut up, however helpful one felt one's contribution or interpretation at that point was going to be. I have found that he was always right. The more important aspect of the situation was never the effect that the analyst's remark was capable of having upon his emotional state, but always the effect of his own free, uninterrupted boldness of expression. What mattered was that he, the patient, was emotionally free to give vent to his thoughts and feelings. If he could do that, the analyst could do nothing better than a silent acquiescence in, or encouragement of, the process.

But to return to our first interview. It is a little tempting to detail all the ego level questions and matters of interest that arise at a first interview, and perhaps there would be no harm in doing this, provided it were clearly understood that this is not analysis, rather the contrary.

From the analyst's point of view, the compilation of a case paper is little different from that outlined under the 'Psychiatric Interview.' He would like information about almost all the same matters: family history, going back in detail to the second or third generation, as well as collaterals. This has more bearing than is generally recognized upon the aetiology of psycho-neurotic troubles. I remember the occasion when I first saw an enormous family tree of the Dusseldorf 'monster.' It seemed to me, on Mendelian laws alone, that it was inevitable that such a pathological individual should spring from all those manifold and various psychopathic ancestors. Similarly, the analyst also wants to know the personal history, with just as much detail, or more, about birth and infancy. Analysis shows us that there can hardly be a severe psychoneurosis without there having been a previous, often equivalent, infantile neurosis.

History-of-the-present-illness draws our attention to pre-cipitating factors. In the field of psychoneurosis, perhaps more than in any other, details of the sexual development are surprisingly constantly amongst the most relevant of all information which we can acquire. Their omission through forgetfulness (possibly repression on the part of the interviewer) has often left one at a loss to understand the case, a loss which has instantly received immediate amendment on the patient's answering almost the first question. This happens time and again.

However, perhaps this more than the other material, with the possible exception of infantile neuroses, is a matter which will not be lost to us if the patient embarks upon a course of analysis, for, sooner or later, his associations of thought will unearth every ascertainable bit of material, and more in the fullness of time.

There are one or two things belonging to reality levels which are best mentioned at a first interview, though it is often very difficult indeed to work them in with our pre-occupation with psychological and emotional values. On this account I sometimes leave them until the interview is over, though, from a time-table point of view, this is not always very practicable.

One is, of course, the subject of fees, and the other, equally important, is the principle of hiring one's time, with the understanding that this should be paid for, whether a patient keeps the appointment or not. Experience teaches us that it is best to arrange for fifty minute sessions at a first interview, otherwise the patient assumes that the sessions are sixty minutes, and it is impossible to keep regular hourly appointment times on such a basis.

The broaching of these matters may lead the patient to ask us a whole series of questions, the number of which can be legion, but perhaps the constant and inevitable one is, 'How long will the treatment last?' There is only one possible answer to this, and that is that we do not know. We may add that the patient is, of course, free to discontinue at any time, preferably with at least a week's notice, but that he should, out of fairness to himself, as well as the analyst, give it at least an eight weeks' run before coming to any conclusion.

The main point at an analytical first interview is to get the patient's transference. Therefore, all these ego matters are of relatively little importance. What is of importance is that he should like coming to see us, or more specifically that he should come again. The best way to achieve this end is to listen to him with sympathy and understanding if he is forthcoming, and to deal with any inhibitions or difficulties which stand in the way of his being forthcoming.

The truth is that before we can affect a person in *any way*, we must win him. The process may be compared to our familiar 'technique' with infants. We do not win the baby or infant by vexing it with anything comparable to 'silly' questions for instance. We aim at giving it a feeling of security, friendliness, and confidence in us. Sometimes we find we can achieve this best by not paying too much obvious attention. When it shows sufficient courage to give expression to itself, then we respond, and, if necessary, encourage. It is something like the process of wooing, though, of course, with adults our 'wooing' must be under the cloak of a purely ego relationship. It must have due regard for their ego defences. Adults will not be so easily 'hoodwinked' as children, though I believe that even children are not continually hoodwinked; that is to say, that if we do not love them, sooner or later our absence of love, or, our hate, will reveal itself, and immediately their defences are erected against us, perhaps permanently. In other words, to succeed consistently, we must be genuine. It is a tremendous effort to act a false part. In time it may become an intolerable effort, and, therefore, for our success, as well as for theirs, deception is not worthwhile. We should be genuine in our liking of the person, and in our desire to help him. If we do not feel this genuine desire, it would be better to send him to another analyst; and if we do not feel it for a sufficient number of people, it would be better that we should not be an analyst.

On the other hand, if we feel that our affective response for the person is too strong to enable us to remain naturally in the position of master of the situation, then, too, perhaps we should get out of it before it has developed. It may be that we ourselves require some more analysis. Even if we can successfully resist positive tendencies towards the patient, we may find that we are doing so by means of a persistent counter resistance. This equally may make us powerless to use the analytical instrument successfully.

I find it impossible to explain how utterly hopeless the average unanalysed person would be in trying to conduct even an analytical interview, leave alone an analysis. We can imagine that every move of his would be likely to be incorrect. He would probably either respond emotionally ('enter the dog fight'), or be utterly and hopelessly repressive ('stopping the dog fight'). It is as though he could not bear the anxiety of watching the phenomenon without doing something one way or the other about it. Not only would the novice be hopeless as an interviewer, but one knows only too well how 'hopeless' he can be in the irresponsible role of an interviewed or prospective patient. He presents himself to the analyst, even at the interview, full of what are obviously the most absurd childish fears and inhibitions, unable to do anything about them, except to take them deadly seriously, terrified of all the infantile and actually harmless bogies in his unconscious mind.

We cannot call his attention to these things. The technique would not work that way. We have to endure with infinite patience such hopeless company! Perhaps that is the art of analysis. We must forego any personal satisfaction or relief. It is not for us to tell him anything. However, in the fullness of time, we have the satisfaction of seeing him in our anxiety-free presence gradually gain courage, and eventually gain such insight and understanding that he can even laugh at what previously frightened him. But this will probably not be for a very considerable time.

A patient who had made some progress and achieved a certain amount of insight, complained to me of the 'unanalysed' society in which he had to live and have his being. He said: 'I am resisting because you are trying to sell me these universal cultural values which I can now see are only symbols and substitutes. I never did like them or respond to them, and analysis has now shown me why. They are not what I wanted; they are 'fob-offs', the things that father and society tried to get me to accept in place of the gratifications I really wanted. Now you are doing it. It is an insult to my intelligence. I will not adapt myself to an ignorant, and what I would call a neurotic, society; moreover, one that has not a vestige of insight into its own neurosis. At least I have got that.

'The structure of Society, its values and beliefs, are a neurosis; and you are asking me to accept that neurosis in place of my own! I suppose *you* would say that we have to accept it, or adapt ourselves to it and manipulate it, without becoming neurotic ourselves. Well, I don't yet know how much I can tolerate of it.'

These remarks suggest that analysts are engaged in unrepressing the 'victims of their own neurosis' (patients) *within* what might be called 'The Social Neurosis.' At any rate analysts have the pleasure of seeing their patients becoming unrepressed and increasingly interesting . . . even if some of these patients do complain that they are having an unanalysed, neurotic, and relatively uninteresting world foisted upon them!

CHAPTER XII

THE ANALYTICAL INTERVIEW
[CONTINUED]

ITS EMOTIONAL BASIS

THE essential ingredient of technique, to which I drew attention in the last chapter, was that of facilitating at the first interview the patient's free and uninhibited expression of himself, all his complaints, his worries, his reasons for coming to see us, his thoughts and fears, theories, hopes, his past, his present, his future prospects, and everything he thought and felt—indeed, everything that was him. The analyst's duty or technique was simply to endeavour to remove any obstacle to this free expression on the part of the patient. The analyst's endeavour may have to go a stage further than hitherto suggested.

For instance, as I have previously indicated instead of the usual immediate outpourings, we frequently get a patient who begins with silence. He seems to be expectant, waiting, perhaps sitting and staring at us. It may be that he is, as it were, in the presence of 'reality', conceding the first move to his august superior. On the other hand he may be just exercising the familiar caution of trying to reassure himself regarding the character and nature of the man he is proposing to confide in. It is not unnatural for one who has still a good deal of ego to do this, before taking the enormous step of plunging into things, and revealing the treasure of his human soul, everything that is precious to him as an individual, the very foundation of his being. This attitude should have our understanding and sympathy.

Whatever his silence is indicating, the practical matter of the moment is to set him at his ease. Everything else can wait. We can bide our time to discover the springs of his taciturnity. How are we to set him at his ease? It will probably require a temporary suspension of our desire to be the passive observer and recipient of his confidences. It will probably require that we immediately become the active (*not too active*), leader of the situation. We offer him a comfortable chair, pray him to be seated, and, unhurriedly but without undue delay, proceed to ask him the usual mundane questions, name, address, age, occupation, civil state, how it came about that he elected to see us, and so on.

This gives him time to mobilize his composure, or reduce his anxiety. Superficially it gives him some reassuring knowledge of us, and it has a generally reassuring effect. Simplicity itself! It is the practical equivalent of the familiar social gambit, weather talk, etcetera, without being so obviously irrelevant. Thus, it is better than social talk, which might indicate to him that we were too much aware of his discomfort and were going out of our way to cover it up. The simplest moves are often the most subtle. The criterion for us to observe is not only that we say nothing to prejudice or to colour or direct the subsequent freedom of the patient, and the natural expression of his true self, particularly as regards the subsequent transference situation. A mere documentary questionnaire will probably not do this. Its chief utility at the opening of an interview for what may become an analysis, is to give the patient time to feel easy, and confiding. But we must remember all the time that our object in the interview is to make the patient feel more at ease, better and happier to be with us, than to give ourselves the satisfaction of a compendious case sheet.

The patient, silent or otherwise, need never be harried. It is best to let his mind work in its own way, but, of course, it would be inadvisable to allow him to go through the appointed hour without telling us as much as possible of the causes which brought him to make an appointment. If he is silent in spite of our indirect casual methods, we may eventually have to give him more direct encouragement. And at a first interview we are naturally justified, if necessary, in appealing to his ego. He made the appointment. Had not he better make the best use of it? And, if he still does not do so, can he say anything about what is holding him back?

However, such difficulties are the exception, and not the rule at a first interview. Initial difficulties in no wise indicate that the patient's analysis will not be as successful as that of the patient who is volubility itself, but suddenly comes to a stop when his pre-conscious material is exhausted, and he meets the inevitable resistance between his conscious and unconscious levels.

However, I would like to suggest that the ideal instrument for analysis is something more than technique. Even insight and the capacity to suppress one's own inappropriate reactions, without feeling too much strain in the process, are not enough. Nothing which the ego can do by itself is enough, though, admittedly, it must have charge of the situation. Perhaps this is what we mean when we call analysis an art. It is that some contribution, the essential contribution, from some part of us that is deeper than the ego, must have a very considerable influence in the situation. The 'id' is *more* than the scientific, more than ego, far more. So many factors enter automatically into the 'id' situation, so many responses and reactions participate naturally and automatically, that science could not assess them, or a fraction of them. Perhaps it is comparable to the very compendious 'technique' which would comprise the ideal, mental form of wooing. Perhaps there are physiological reactions (there are), that count for more than the psychological ones—certainly for more than the conscious ones. It goes without saying that no negative affects enter into it. Is it ever adequate for the ego to take over what the id does so naturally and easily? In my opinion it is not, not in our present state of scientific knowledge. Would it ever be? Bearing in mind that the unconscious (the part which counts) relationship of the interviewed to the interviewer is on an id level, and its effects are comparable to those of being wooed, will it ever respond to an ego technique?

I feel that I must here illustrate my point with an analytical story, which, incidentally, helps to show the frequent uselessness of case sheet material elicited at a first interview. In answer to direct questions, a woman patient informed me that her relationship with her husband was everything that could be desired, 'perfect.' I had asked her the questions because the nature of the phobias from which she suffered, and her general state of acute anxiety neurosis, suggested a disordered sexual life.

Very soon she brought me a dream in which a large bird had flown over her prostrate body, and had touched her with the tip of one of its wings. This was the climax to what amounted to a nightmare, and she awoke screaming. In association of thought, she screamed again! She said, with hysterical emphasis, 'It's my husband. When he touches me, I want to scream. I try not to; I stifle it. The trouble, doctor, is this: He means well, but he hasn't a clue about how to make love or sex to a woman. What makes it

worse is that the poor fellow tries his best. He is an intelligent
man, and he reads up everything on the subject. I have read the
blessed books too. Whatever he tries to do to me, I could almost
tell him the page of Havelock Ellis from which he has learned it.
I think I shall go mad if he does not leave me alone. Yet I can't
tell him this. He means to try so hard, and it would hurt him too
much.'

In short, this husband's ego was trying to take on by the exercise
of a technique, a function which his id should have been doing
quite naturally and effortlessly. His id was obviously impotent,
but all the efforts of his ego to amend this by ego-potency were
obviously doing more harm than good. Far from having a gratifying effect upon his partner in the sexual 'interview', it was
having very much the opposite effect. I am tempted to ask if *you*
would entertain a relationship, even a conversation, with a person,
friend or otherwise, whom you knew to be trying his technique
on you!

Now, in so far as the effects we have upon others in personal
interviews, however camouflaged, under ego auspices, are unconscious and fundamentally unconsciously emotional, be they
instinct or art, no ego system of technique in analysis is going to
be an adequate substitute for the mental 'wooing', the success
of which will alone be success indeed.

Here an equally important matter deserves our consideration
before we close the subject of the analytical interview: when we
have been successful in our mental 'wooing' of the person, will
we *want* the responsibility that the consequent situation places
upon us? The responsibility is that of, in due course, 'educating'
him, modifying him. It entails, amongst other things, disciplining
him. We have undertaken a very responsible job, for, as with
children our objective is education. It is more than education; it
is deep-seated modification (e.g. sublimation) in gratification,
though our task will not be complete until he is well enough to
negotiate his own gratification. The question for us is: 'Will our
total psyche be equal to the task?' If we doubt it, we should not
begin.

Here I feel I must add a most important rider, in case of mis-
understanding. I must emphasize that anything approaching
education or modification of a patient should not be attempted,

not in the slightest degree, until the full transference stage of analysis has been established. At first interviews, and, in fact, throughout the early stages of analysis, we should be wary of saying anything except for the sole purpose of removing resistance to the patient's free association of thought and analytical progress. I have usually found it inadvisable even to interpret dreams. Just let the patient talk, doing free association of thought, and so long as he is making analytical progress, be content. Do not let even his silences provoke anxiety in you, or you will fail to deal with them appropriately. One's business is to understand this and any other resistance, even the over-talkative one, that may be impeding the analytical movement; and, having understood it, to remove it by interpretation.

In other words, during the early stages of analysis, indeed right up to the full development of transference, the analyst is concerned only with the removal of resistances to analytical progress. This includes, of course, keeping the patient at his ease. It is practically always anxiety which acts as a resistance barrier. This must be appropriately interpreted at the right moment, when it is impeding progress.

Do not attempt to teach the patient, or to correct, or to undeceive. By this I do not mean that one should actively support his mistakes or illusions. I mean merely that to try to teach or to correct tends to cause him to react to it as to emotional opposition (e.g. hate), and to arouse his resistance. He will learn more if resistance is dissipated, and free association and analytical progress continued. In fact, this is the only way he will learn anything. To this end also, one should be wary of saying anything, however wise or true, that the patient may have difficulty in believing. As his mind, through this process of free association and removal of resistance to free association, proceeds, transference will develop. Its development may cause a special form of crisis of its own. Sooner or later its presence must be brought to consciousness, whether it has revealed itself or not.

Those who have been inadequately analysed will probably be afraid of transference, will be afraid to bring the discussion to a personal emotional level between the patient and themselves. I venture to say that until this is done, and until the patient has gained a sufficient sense of security and courage to say, and to keep on saying, his personal feelings, however personal both to himself and the analyst, the process of analysis proper has not been fully established. I would go further and say that unless the analyst is able to receive both the patient's positive (love) feelings, and also his vituperations and hate, however cleverly directed and near to the mark, without himself being aroused to any emotional response whatsoever, transference analysis will not be taking place.

It is necessary that the analyst should be able to recognize immediately all these declarations and expostulations on the part of the patient, as a reliving of the patient's infantile amnesia—his forgotten repressed emotional relationship towards his parents in infancy—before he is competent to complete the analytical process. The analyst must be so familiar with the phenomenon of people reliving their Oedipus complex and assigning to him the role in it of loved and hated parent, that he is in no danger whatsoever of accepting their love-and-hate (however aptly directed) at its face value. More than this: the analyst must here be on such familiar ground, by virtue both of his own personal analysis and his daily and hourly insight into a succession of patients, that he instantly knows, without doubt or hesitation, that all their feelings and phantasies and rationalizations, everything they express in regard to himself, are nothing more or less than the old Oedipus drama being relived, re-experienced and dramatized afresh. Further, he must have full insight into similar tendencies in himself, and be able to discount them entirely. All this is a necessary prerequisite for his appropriate handling of the situation.

CHAPTER XIII

ANALYSIS—RESISTANCE AND
TECHNIQUE

W E should not try to persuade a person to be analysed. If a psychiatrist or analyst is indicated, no more is required than that the sufferer should be put in touch with him. There should be no agenda, nothing on the programme, except the one consultation, the one interview. Everything hangs upon this. Indeed, the interview, the first interview, is of such great importance, whether it be a new doctor, a general practitioner, psychiatrist, or analyst, that I am making it the main subject matter of this book.

The issue is not whether to be analysed, or not to be analysed. The issue is not whether analysis is a good thing or a bad thing, whether its tenets are true or false, whether it makes people better or worse, or anything of that sort. The issue is simply whether you are troubled in mind or body, and whether you would like to consult someone whose business it is to help those who are in the sort of trouble you are in.

The interview may last five minutes, an hour, or a succession of hours, a day, a week, a month, or a year. In any case, its importance cannot be over-estimated. Most people, if in trouble, or at any rate if their trouble threatens to become greater than they can bear, naturally look for help, like the babes and children they once were, and still are. They wish to find the good parent-surrogate to put everything right for them as mother used to do in childhood.

To be worthy of the role assigned him, and competent to handle it, particularly in the deep waters of what I have called the 'year-long interview', the analyst must be a person who has become familiar with his own unconscious complexes and anxieties, who has laid all the ghosts or bogies in his own unconscious, and is no longer afraid of them. The analyst must be free from anxiety himself, free from fear of the unconscious mind, both his own and the patient's; and this freedom from fear must be based upon a familiar and conscious intimacy with all that exists, and can possibly exist, within.

Unfortunately, the analyst is usually the very last person consulted, and then only when everything else and everybody else have failed. Unanalysed people, placed by the despairing sufferer, clutching at the first straw, in the responsible role of parent-figure or analyst, will practically always support the defensive and resistant forces (super-ego) in the sufferer's mind *against* even legitimate and practicable tendencies to tension reduction and instinct relief. That is to say, they will encourage defences, encourage resistances. They will act as super-egos. They will take-on, too literally perhaps, the role of the harsh or oppressive parent who may well have been the original cause of all the trouble. That is to say, their 'treatment', unless they are very exceptional, may well prove to be the antithesis of analysis. Probably they will not do much harm, because, at the very best, both patient and 'therapist' will be confining their attention and discourse only to manifestations on a conscious level, and will be quite unaware of the real forces involved, of the real sources both of the distress, and even of the improvement that may temporarily ensue. The benefits derived are likely to be superficial, temporary, and transient, and ultimately inadequate. They will be due to causes (transference mechanisms) of which neither party will have the slightest cognizance.

Like the layman, doctor, and psychiatrist, the analyst also is interested in manifestations, and in what he and other medical men would call 'symptomatology'. But symptoms, no matter how plentiful, do not in themselves constitute the disease, or, necessarily, tell us its nature, source and origin—the sort of knowledge we require to get at its roots, and put it right.

Psychiatrists, having frequently to deal with massive disorders, the psychological manifestations of which are commonly very severe, often tend to become interested in the chemical, physical, or physiological accompaniments, hoping to find a clue to the disturbance at such a basic level as that. There would appear to be much justification for such a research, despite its sterility so far, for it is rare to find mental illness without some physical counterpart, or physical illness without mental changes.

The psychological or analytical point of view may be said to be that our adaptation to environment is primarily a psychological one, and that the spearhead, as it were, of adaptations or changes within us is connected with psychological motivations. In short, if we are unfrustrated psychologically, there is, in practice, little cause for anything to go wrong. The analytical theory of psychological motivation is essentially a dynamic one, based upon instinctual drives, infantile emotional reactive patterns, and indeed, all our unconscious strivings and fears influencing the conscious level of the mind. In addition to reality, there are also psychological forces frustrating or inhibiting the natural gratification of instincts and impulses. These psychological frustrators often prove to be more effective than reality, though certainly less necessary. Our conscious will is found to be more a product of them, of the frustrating forces, than it is an instrument of the unconscious instinct-drives which really empower the essential movements of our lives.

Now, as I have said, though the analyst is interested, like everybody else, in manifestations, his particular characteristic is that he is even more interested in what is not manifest, in what lies behind the manifestations. To him the manifestations are of interest chiefly as a clue to the unconscious processes that determine them. Even at such a simple interview as the therapeutic one, which I have described, there is a great deal going on that is not apparent on the surface. And it is this more than anything conscious or apparent which produces the results, both morbid and symptomatic, and therapeutic and beneficial. Therefore, it is worthy of our attention.

For instance while the patient is telling the therapist her secrets, unconscious mental operations are going on in her, and if it were not for these the process would do her no good. Emotions that were pent-up, and attached to the subject matter of her story, have for many years been held back, partly even from her own conscious considerations. She has been struggling to repress them, and, in consequence, has been suffering tension unrelieved. By virtue of putting the analyst, in this case particularly as he was a stranger, in the place of a good parent-image, she was able to gain sufficient courage, sufficient freedom from fear, to allow these ghosts or bogies to emerge more freely to the surface, thereby discharging some of her pent-up tension, which she would otherwise have been afraid to discharge in its entirety.

Also she was probably managing to make the analyst take the place of her super-ego, so that he was endowed by her with, as it were, powers of forgiveness, something approaching omnipotence. It was through unconscious mechanisms of this nature that she felt so relieved, so much better after the interview. The analyst should be aware of all this, and, therefore, in a position to use this knowledge if it is required, as will be the case if the interview proceeds to a deeper level of analysis.

Also during the interview there is something going on in the analyst. Otherwise he would not be interested in being an analyst. It is even more especially his business to know exactly what is going on within himself. If he did not know, he would be apt to assume the role, however absurd, assigned to him by the patient. He might even pose as a professional wise man, as an infallible adviser, or even as a deity. Knowing himself as he does, he is able to deal with and treat the patient and the situation objectively, and not to fall into the trap of assuming the role assigned to him. For instance, he will not react to love by giving love, nor to hate by giving hate, but will, under all circumstances, remain the physician whose object it is to benefit the persons consulting him by eventually revealing them—that is to say, their resistance, and their unconscious mind—to themselves, and putting their own ego in charge of their emotions and of their situation. In short, it is only by virtue of his insight into himself, and into the patients, that he is secure from entering what I have called the 'dog-fight' with them. It is this as much as anything else that qualifies him for the role, the role which unanalysed persons are most unlikely to fill satisfactorily, apart from the most superficial aspects of it.

What I am trying to emphasize in this chapter is that, whereas we normally concentrate our attention upon manifestations or symptoms, and confine our attention to these, the analyst is interested in them chiefly in so far as they are clues to something that is going on incessantly in the unconscious mind. Whether it is the symptoms, for instance, of psychoneurotic illness, whether it is dreams, phantasies, or hypnagogic hallucinations (which we can most of us see if we are very tired or sleepy and close our eyes), everything that moves us in thought and deed to life, to death, or to reproduction, is a manifestation of something that is going on continually in the deeper or unconscious level of the mind.

Therapeutic measures in the analytical sense must be directed towards this material, and the first step is, of course, to enable it to enter consciousness, because it is only when it is on a conscious plane that we can do anything about it. It is only there that the conscious ego can have any say in the matter.

Now it may well be asked, 'What *is* it that goes on? Why don't you, or any other analyst, simply tell us what it is?' The reason is that if I told you at this stage you would immediately fling me and my book as far away from you as possible! The truth is that what goes on in the repressed unconscious is everything that you resist, repudiate, and deny.

It is not the technique of analysis, at least not of psycho-analysis, to *tell* resisted unconscious material. Such a procedure, in as much as it would only increase the resistances, would be the very antithesis of psycho-analysis. The technique of psycho-analysis, and do not forget it, is to remove, to interpret the *resistances*. And we might say throughout the first stage of analysis the technique is pretty well confined to that. At a first interview we generally do not go so far as that. Even most of the resistances have unfortunately to be left intact. In general it can be said that it is only by the removal, through interpretation, of resistances that analysis has discovered what it is that is being resisted. When a resistance is removed, that modicum of resisted material is ready to emerge to a conscious level. In any case, only then would it have any *meaning* for us. Generally speaking, we either get the emotions welling-up without the material, or if we get the material, we do not get the relevant emotions that, in the unconscious, belong to it. As a result it has no *meaning* for us. The 'meaning' of things is an emotional experience. Life itself has no 'meaning' if we feel nothing.

In a sense I could tell you some of the things in the unconscious, but they would be meaningless—or their meaning would be hotly denied. As I have said, they include everything that is censored and abhorred and feared. It is this very repudiation that has repressed all these primitive things into what is called the repressed unconscious. It is not only murder, rape, and all the perversions, but even cannibalism! You cannot *feel* this; therefore you cannot know its meaning. Ernest Jones says it can be summed up in two words : "incest and murder." (*Papers on P-A.*, p. 359).

But to say all this is not analytical or psycho-analytical. Analysis is primarily concerned with our *resistances* to knowing, through intrusion into consciousness, what lies beneath consciousness. Anyone who is afraid of his own unconscious material cannot hope to make a patient or analysand unafraid, any more than a child who is afraid of the dark can hope to make another fearful child unafraid of it. The blind cannot lead the blind successfully, nor the fearful lead others to fearlessness.

Now this brings us to the principal operation of the first stage of analysis. It can be summarized by saying our business throughout the first stage is almost confined to removing resistances, analysing them, and interpreting them if necessary—resistances to free association of thought, resistances to the progress of the analytical movement. In due course this will lead us to the so-called second stage, during which the patient is unwittingly reliving his childhood, or infantile emotional life, with the analyst in the role which his parents or parent-surrogates once occupied. At that stage the analyst interprets everything freely, but the important point is, he certainly does not do so until that stage has arrived. What started as an interview has reached a very different level when we come to transference, transference resistance, and transference interpretation.

To summarize: one might say that the chief characteristics of analytical technique, particularly in the case of psycho-analysis, are: one, a degree of *passivity* on the part of the analyst incredible to anyone who has not experienced it; two, the consistent application of the basic rule, namely the principle of *free association of thought*; and, three, the interpretation in the early stages of little else except *resistances*, or anything which impedes the progress and development of the analytical movement.

Even more characteristic than any of these is, of course, the underlying movement which has been called *the strategic development of the transference*. Analysis proper may be said to consist in the appropriate dealing with the transference, particularly, exposure of it, and free interpretation of it once it has been established.

In spite of this stereotyped outline, most people would agree that the personality of the analyst does inevitably enter into the situation. I would go further, and suggest that each analyst has, to some extent, his own technique. Some are probably more technical than others. It is about as difficult to describe techniques as it would be to explain how to make friends and influence people. They are not things that one can do exclusively with one's ego or conscious will. They are best done naturally (though it is surprising how little 'nature' enters into the technique of some analysts). As I suggested in a previous chapter: imagine conversing socially with a man who is trying his technique on you! Probably in ten minutes you would have found him out, and in another ten you would want to get away from him. He would be an insufferable bore, except to people who are easily taken in. The practice of psychology should be the very antithesis of taking people in. Its purpose is to expose cant and deception, to remove defences and reticence, and to reveal the naked truth . . . in so far as our dim eyes can bear to see it.

I have suggested that there may be as many techniques as there are analysts, though the basic principles may be common to all— one essential is that of not intruding or attempting initial modification of the patient's 'errors' before transference is established. I have suggested also that there are probably as many techniques, at any rate at first interviews, as there are patients. We all of us intuitively recognize that we must adjust our contact with any person we meet, according to the psychology of that person; and this we do at first interviews also, whether we know we are doing it or not. We do not beat our head against a stone wall; experience, if nothing else, will soon teach us that some of our patients' psyches are as unmodifiable as the proverbial stone wall. We find we must let them express their own thoughts, emotions and theories, however nonsensical (generally they are more 'sensible' than sense), otherwise we will only arouse their resistance and increase our difficulties in getting anywhere with them, or getting them anywhere.

Although each patient may require a technique appropriate to his particular psychology, sometimes a very simple or even a slightly psychotic psychology, it is as well for the operator to be able to do major surgery, even if the particular operation he is called upon to perform is often quite a little one. No operation, however small, is an insignificant matter to the patient.

I now propose to give a few illustrative analytical interviews, beginning with an unusually simple one. Although these case-papers may fail to illustrate a great many of the principles that have been discussed, there is at least one thing which most of them will illustrate, namely, the truth of my statement that we are all resistant to what lies in our repressed unconscious. And this naturally applies to the analyst as much as to the patient, except in so far as the former has achieved some release from his repressions.

PARTS III TO V: PRACTICE

PART THREE
THE INTERVIEWED

FROM THEORY TO PRACTICE

CHAPTER XIV

A CASE OF BLUSHING

THE first case I shall describe is a particularly simple one. It will be seen that although the interview proceeded with apparent smoothness, technical difficulties, especially as regards therapy, were practically insuperable at first. Had this patient been capable of insight without treatment, it may be that he could not have developed his particular symptoms.

He was a single young man, very tense and awkward, whose complaint can be put under the familiar category of *blushing*, though in his case blushing had developed a very peculiar and interesting form of expression.

In spite of his embarrassment, or because of it, he lost no time in plunging into his story: 'I have always been very nervous and self-conscious, but the trouble has been getting worse for some months. It used to be *blushing*, very severe, getting all hot and flushed, breaking into a sweat; but, lately (you may think it very stupid), it has developed into something quite intolerable, quite impossible—I have thought of throwing up my job, and clearing out of the country; I just can't stand it going on while I am at work. Before this last thing developed there was no crazy idea; I was just nervous, inclined to blush, very uncomfortable; but now it is this thing that I can't stand.'

He paused. I sat there looking blank and stupid. At length I asked, 'What is it?'

'What is it?' He expostulated, 'Can't you see what it is? It is my *ear* burning and going red. I thought of throwing up my work, because it's worse in the office. All the time at work I am in a continual fear of it happening . . .'

Analyst: 'Perhaps that's what brings it on?'

'Yes, yes, you are right, I suppose it is the fear of it happening that actually brings it on.'

As, at this point, he was a little dumb, I asked another question. He replied: 'Yes, there is a girl at the office. She sits opposite me. She's a peculiar girl, only about nineteen, but I know she is continually looking at me. I don't feel too good about it, because I realize that this red ear may come on at any moment, and I shall feel awful, and want to chuck up the whole job, and get out. I think she realizes that my ear sticks out too much at this spot, and that it is abnormal. She gives me the impression that she is looking at it. All the time I feel that the ear-burning is going to come on, and I shall be noticed; she will notice it. I find it difficult to go to work on account of this fear. I breathe a sigh of relief when the day is over.'

The reader may, by this time, have suspected that, while this was the current, conscious form of this young man's morbid anxiety and worry, it had had a history, an antecedent, which was now less acutely conscious, perhaps partly repressed. This antecedent was the familiar, protracted pubertal and post-pubertal period of masturbation with worry, undue fear of it, and unsuccessful attempts to suppress it.

It is not always a good thing to ask a patient to detail his masturbation phantasy at any time in analysis, particularly at a first interview, but somehow it emerged in this instance. It was a pretty normal one, namely that of unclothing in imagination some member of the opposite sex. He had never actually experienced any sexual intercourse. The matters of special psychological interest were, one, that for some years masturbation had in his opinion been excessive, two, that a development of his phantasy had been the unclothing of, and imaginary intercourse with, the particular girl who sat opposite him at the office, and, three, most relevant of all, the fact that he had, in recent months, succeeded, by dint of great struggle and effort, in relatively suppressing these thoughts and activities; with the result, he said, that they now occurred only once in two or three weeks. Asked for the reason of this he said simply: 'The reason I have not done it more often is that I don't think I should.'

The psychopathology of his symptom can, therefore, be outlined as follows. His sexual instincts, at puberty and after puberty, had met with the familiar frustrations, inhibitions and attempts at repression. A conflict had been set up between instinct on the one hand, and super-ego ('I don't think I should'), plus ego, on the other hand, with the result that sexual tendencies had been suppressed, and, to some extent, repressed. The girl who sits opposite him at work acts as a stimulus to both sides of this semi-repressed conflict. On the one hand, she stands for the imaginary gratification, and, on the other hand, more consciously, she stands for the reproving super-ego, prohibiting any such thoughts, creating feelings of guilt at having indulged in them, and causing consequent anxiety, suppressed anger and discomfort. The unconscious repressed guilt with its attendant threats of punishment, and unconscious castration anxiety, need not here be stressed, except to remind us that the *anxiety* at least breaks through repression and emerges into consciousness as a symptom. The effect of all this is that tumescence, sexual or genital tumescence, is effectively inhibited. He is not now conscious of any feelings of sexuality towards the girl. He is conscious only of the opposite, namely of anxiety and discomfort.

The tendency to tumescence which, in the absence of conflict, would have been experienced genitally, is strong enough to have escaped from repression by the familiar mechanism of displacement. Previously, in its first displacement, it expressed itself in his symptom of blushing, his face 'hot, flushed and sweating.' There is probably also a reaction of anger at frustration, lending a physiological basis to the humerous expression, 'was my face red!' At the same time, this symptom implemented the exposure and the punishment which his super-ego would inflict upon him for the guilty tumescence. With the further development of this illness, the tumescence has found a more specific phallic symbol for its expression and for his exposure, namely, his ear.

This case, though very obvious and superficial, may be of some interest as representing in a rather more severe form than usual the very familiar, almost universal, mechanisms of shyness and blushing.

I should add that, in this patient's case, morbidity went a little deeper, and was rather more severe, than our discussion hitherto reveals. It transpired that the part of his projecting outer ear, or pinna, on which his guilty and discomforting thoughts were concentrated, was the little protuberance in front of the aperture, called the tragus. He had what might almost be called 'ideas of reference' associated with this. He actually half-believed the following phantastic story.

He said: 'Some months ago I had an accident when mountaineer-

D

ing. I fell and rolled down what was almost a precipice. I do not know if the sticking out of this part of my ear was the result of the fall, but I have noticed it only subsequent to the fall.' He was facing me at the time, and I pointed out to him that his other ear was exactly the same, quite symmetrical. He said: 'Yes, I know they are exactly the same on both sides,' rather impatiently, as though this fact were an unnecessary interference with the phantasy or delusion which he wished to maintain in reference to his left ear only. It was this ear which was nearer the girl who sat almost, but not quite, opposite him at the office; it was this ear only which was in the habit of becoming red and burning. He went on to tell me how various people had pointed out to him the prominence of this part of his ear, or at least 'indicated' that they had noticed it. He said: 'I have only to look in the mirror now, and it makes me feel abnormal and ashamed.' It is possible that the opening or 'ear-hole', immediately behind the tragus, made this visible part of his anatomy more accurately symbolical of the secret part which shame must conceal.

I do not think that it is a very far cry from the shame, from the feeling of abnormality now concentrated upon his ear, or this particular part of his ear, to the equivalent feelings of shame and abnormality which obsessed him during the early years of his masturbatory compulsion and conflict. However, the tendency to such ideas as these later ones, puts a graver aspect to the case. It suggests a slightly schizoid element, with a leaning towards paranoid ideas of reference. The rest of his psychopathology might be regarded as psychoneurotic, but this latter aspect suggests the admixture of a psychotic trend.

However, I am inclined to say that, in the absence of a family history of any important mental illness, in the absence of any marked infantile neurosis, and any previous mental breakdown, the prognosis in this case is probably quite good. Many of us pass through not only psychoneurotic but even tentative, mild, or borderline psychotic trends, and develop away from them rather than into them.

From the point of view of technique at a first interview, one may say that the confession of all these things to me, particularly the spontaneous confession of a good deal of his sexual life, indicates the lifting of some resistances, and would tend to initiate the development of some transference. In so far as he is rather more the schizoid than the hysterical type, that initial transference will be small. Nevertheless, it may prove the starting point towards a relationship which would have enabled me to help him, had the opportunity presented itself. I venture to think that had I attempted interpretation of his symptom, such for instance as telling him, this particular repressed young man, that the symptom meant nothing more or less than that he was automatically using his ear as a phallic symbol (and thereby playing into the hands of his castrating superego and ego), all I would have achieved is a checking of the transference tendency to me, and, perhaps, through me, to any subsequent psychotherapist. At least I think I avoided increasing his resistances.

I am sorry to say that circumstances (my time-table) were such that I had to transfer him elsewhere for treatment; but I think we can have hopes of a great deal of amelioration, particularly when his sexual life achieves its expression in more normal, ego-syntonic ways.

CHAPTER XV

ACTING OUT OUR CONFLICTS

CASE

NOT every patient presents himself complaining of symptoms which are recognizable as such. A good many people, as mentioned in a previous chapter, appear to be the victims of misfortune or 'malignant fate'. Anyhow, things have not gone right with them, through no fault of their own—or at least through no very apparent fault. It is sad to say that such appearances practically always reveal themselves as rationalizations or defences against the recognition of deep-seated complexes or morbid trends, which the unfortunate victim is unconsciously acting out, dramatizing, and thereby making his distress appear to be due to external or real causes, when it is actually due to internal ones.

Naturally the victims of such symptomatic behaviour do not immediately complain to a psychologist, or present themselves for treatment. They try to 'put things right' by manipulating reality, by various activities in their actual life. They never get anywhere with these endeavours because the compulsion to act out their complex is the real driving force. If they do come for analysis (the only process which in these cases will put everything right) it is commonly by some 'accident!' They are not at all ready to believe that their troubles emanate from their own conflicts and complexes. All these characteristics were present in the following case.

She was a woman in the early thirties. She had had a sort of token marriage in her youth. It had never had any real emotional meaning, and after a few useless attempts to make adjustment, the husband had been divorced while she was still very young. Nevertheless, she was a highly cultured, well-educated, and much-travelled lady. It would seem that the one subject she did not know very much about was psychology. There was another subject in which she felt her knowledge inadequate, and that was foreign languages, but she was at present busily engaged in remedying this latter defect.

Unlike most patients that consult one, she appeared to be very much at home from the moment of her arrival. She offered me a cigarette (which I accepted), and threw herself restlessly into a large chair. She announced: 'There is nothing wrong with me, you know!' On my enquiring as to what had induced her to make the appointment, she said: 'Well, I have come to see you for purely emotional reasons.'

She had not expressed her thought very well for what she meant by this was that she had come to see me purely on account of the pressure from a man friend to whom she was emotionally attached, and by whom she was, therefore, at the moment, much influenced. He had, as it were, pushed her into it. She said: 'You see, the man I am interested in at present has been analysed, and it is one of his main interests in life. *He* wanted me to come and see you. He is mad on everybody getting analysed.'

What all this meant, so it transpired, was that her man friend had broken off his analysis very prematurely, and had since been busy offering everybody he met to analysis as vicarious sacrifices in lieu of himself, who, it seemed, really needed it most. I thought this was such a bad beginning, such a bad reason for her analysis, that I had little hope at that moment of her proving to be a serious analysand. It is rare for a person pressed by another into an analytical interview to settle down to treatment. He or she is more likely to pay a perfunctory visit, just to prove that the idea was unnecessary or absurd.

However, she reduced my pessimism a little by saying: 'That is one part of my reason for coming to see you.' Naturally, I then asked if she would care to tell me what was the other part of her reason. She said: 'Oh, well, it's just an interest of my own. I felt I'd like to come and see what it is all about. Frankly, I think that all this psychology is a bit of bunk—hooey. But this man I am in love with, or seem to be in love with, is so fantastically keen on it—and he is a very brainy person—so I thought I'd better just come and see.

'Oh, well, I suppose I might as well tell you who he is. He is Signor Don Ferdinand, the celebrity who teaches me Spanish, the subject which I am now studying. Having travelled everywhere and experienced the disadvantage of not knowing the language of

the country I was in well enough, I have now, in my old age (!),
decided to become a linguist.'

At this point, with a little temerity, as it may hardly have been
good technique, I bluntly asked this blunt woman what was her
means of support. She said: 'Oh, I am one of the fortunate ones,
though I wouldn't say that I have no financial worries. In fact,
I did phone a Clinic for the purpose of trying to get analysed
there, but I found they had too long a waiting list; and there are
all sorts of other difficulties.'

'But,' said I, 'It seems that you are not at all sure that you want
analysis?'

'Oh, yes, I have made up my mind; that is why I have come.'

'Why do you want to be analysed?'

'Oh, I suppose it's because I think I'm in love with this man,
and he says I should be analysed. Perhaps I am too easily persu-
aded. But I think there are some other slight little personal things.'

'Such as what?'

'Oh, when I try and do an examination paper, I get in a flap;
and he says analysis will help me to keep calm.'

I then asked her if there were any other slight little personal
things that she would care to tell me. Her attitude to this encouragement might be summed up as, 'What cheek!! Why the
hell should I tell you?' She said, in effect: 'No, there are not: I
don't need to tell you anything. I have nothing to get off my chest.
All this is a lot of hooey anyway. I can manage my own life myself,
thank you very much,' and so forth.

We seemed to be getting nowhere, but I was beginning to
sense something of the emotional nature of the motivations of this
woman; and to sense my tendency to react to them. Contrary to
any prescribed technique, I tried her with a bit of her own emotional
language, expressed, of course, without emotion. I said: 'What
makes you suppose that you are analysable at all?' She was a little
startled, lest it were being alleged that she had the defect of 'not
being analysable.'

She said: 'Do you really mean that? Is that possible?'

I said, 'Well, your tendency seems to be reticent, instead of
forthcoming. You don't seem to want to tell me anything about
yourself. That is all the very antithesis of the desire to be analysed.'

Curiously enough, she seemed a little consoled; she said, 'That's me. I am normally a reticent person.' Then, yielding more to a tendency to warm up to me, she said: 'You see, the truth is, *I don't like* my past life.' After a pause, she added: 'The fact is that I am very happy being in love with Ferdinand, although I have only known him for a few months. I think it is rare for me to be having a happy love affair. Mostly they have been so disastrous. This Spaniard has all the qualities of brain, as well as a magnificent virile body. It is the first really satisfactory and happy love affair which I have had for years. I don't want you or analysis or anything else to mess it up.'

I tried to look sympathetic as she continued: 'My past has been full of unfortunate and unhappy affairs. The men who have loved me, I have usually not loved. I sometimes tried to be kind to them out of sympathy . . . with disastrous effects upon myself. There are still some men wanting to marry me. Two or three have been hanging about for years. (This proved to be true). But I have learned such dreadful lessons that I have a sort of phobia of the approach of any of them. My very first love affair was a sort of minor tragedy. Shall I tell you about it?'

With the prospect of hearing this story, my pessimism regarding this patient's proclivity for analysis, which she obviously needed so badly, turned to optimism. I thought to myself, 'Good gracious, after starting by being so tough, she is now proposing to hand me her heart on a platter.' I felt somehow that that was what she was proposing at that moment.

She told me: 'It was when I was only nineteen years of age. I was a student in Germany. Of course, a certain amount of flirting went on amongst the undergraduates, but nothing of any importance. We knew how to look after ourselves—all a silly lot of boys and girls, and I was far from being in love with any of them. Then, at some dance affair, I met a most splendid looking man. He was about thirty-five. He danced with me, and during that brief evening, I fell for him, hook, line, and sinker. He must have sensed something of my adoration, for at the end he saw me out, and offered to drive me home. I let him. He actually took me up to the place where I was living, and stopped outside. Perhaps I showed some reluctance to leave. Anyhow, the next thing he said to me was: 'It's not very late yet, let me drive you to my flat, and show you my pictures.' It may be difficult for you to understand, but the fact of it was that I was so infatuated with this man that there is absolutely nothing that I would not have done had he asked me. I suppose you will think I was crazy. Perhaps I was. Anyhow, I was so bewildered and confused that I have no clear recollection of anything that happened. He drove me home in the early hours, and I think I must have fallen into a sort of stupor.

'However insane I was at the time, I awoke in full possession of my faculties, painfully sane. I cannot tell you the agonies I passed through, not only that day, and the following night, but all through that week. I told nobody, but I had one of the most acutely painful and miserable weeks of my whole life. I bore it all alone. It was as though something inside me was eating out my heart and soul. Yet —this caps the whole stupid thing—at the end of the week, after all that agony, when this man suddenly popped up again, with the same shocking proposal, I just fell into his arms, as though again I could not help myself. He never believed I was a virgin. Something happened the following week, during my second spell of agony, that steeled my defences against him. It may have been the fact that I learned that he was the most notorious wolf in the neighbourhood; or more likely, it was that something penetrated from him into my thickhead—the awful realization that I meant as little to him as he meant much to me. Anyhow, during that second week, I somehow pulled myself together. He verified my worst fears, for, as soon as I refused him, he dropped me immediately, and never troubled to see me again. What a way to begin the romance of one's love life!'

What a way indeed! But this little story is of considerable psychological interest, because it transpired that throughout her life, right up to this last affair, and her coming to see me, this woman had been engaged in 'symptomatic behaviour' of this sort. This was an example of what might be called the libidinal pattern. In due course she presented me with plenty of examples of the opposite or reactive pattern, one of which was her marriage. It was not difficult to bring to her notice, that she had married the husband she did marry *because* her emotions were not involved! In short, her adult-long succession of examples of symptomatic behaviour, comprising her entire love life, or life of personal relationships, reveals its source in unresolved conflict. The ingredients of this conflict are, on the one hand, sexual impulse and phantasy, alternating, on the other hand, with defences and re-action formations. The dynamic drive of each of these contestants is apparently so great that her ego is, as it were, buffeted about from one camp to the other. Whichever camp it is in, it is subject, sooner or later, to a terrible beating-up by the opposite side. This conflict, making, as it did, for lack of adjustment to reality, in-stability, and alternating episodes of ecstasy and agony, is still there, and still continues to order her conduct, and to express or to dramatize itself in the succession of affairs and resistances right up to date.

I had no doubt that this last affair of hers, the current one, would prove, in these respects, no different from its predecessors—just as symptomatic as the rest. Such a conclusion was plain to me, even without the further knowledge (omitted, perhaps on account of its triviality), that the admirable Spaniard already had a wife and large family, safely housed in Spain.

D•

CHAPTER XVI

THE SEQUEL

THE chief interest in this case, from the point of view of the first interview, was this: Having started by presenting resistances in the form of: 'nothing wrong with me,' a 'purely intellectual curiosity to know what all this hooey is about,' 'I have come in order to please the man who is my lover.' 'Why the hell should I tell you anything about myself?' and so on; and having proceeded to a giving of herself, this time in the form of a recital of her first sexual experience, the recital now developed into an admission of a whole conglomeration of the suspected symptoms which she is busily ignoring. They come out singly, and in bunches, sometimes with flimsy attempts at rationalization. She says, for instance, 'I hope you will not get me wrong—well, I know you won't—when I tell you that I am better when I have a man friend. You see, if I don't have one, or if things are wrong in that department, I take to drinking too much. This frightens me rather because my father used to. I have done that in company too; I have even had an occasional fainting attack at a party; but it's not really heavy drinking. It takes only a little to knock me out, and I feel dreadful all the next day after it. I think I have done it partly through feeling over-exhausted. I must be a bit of a fool; I get caught in so many ways. For instance, I only went to this Spaniard because he is middle-aged, a married man with a family, and I thought that, in consequence, everything would be unemotional. I thought I laid my plans carefully to avoid being caught up in this emotional vortex; and here I am, caught again.'

I feel inclined to dwell upon this subject for a moment as it points to the conflict which lies at the basis of this patient's troubles. The fact is that this woman has a tremendous capacity for transference. Far from being unanalysable, the accusation with which I challenged her in the early stages of her first interview, her nature is such that it impels her compulsively to a transference to somebody—to anybody who is ready to receive it. It is an imperative need of her nature. For a decade or more, the people

ready to receive this transference of hers, the people who have set
out to encourage it, who have made advances to her for this
purpose, have naturally been men who had an emotional axe to
grind. They felt or sensed her need, and felt or sensed their desire
to meet it. It is as though the man's mind, perhaps subconsciously,
felt: 'Here is a woman who needs something, who is hungering
for something. I can use her'—though perhaps they would not
all admit to thoughts quite in that conscious form.

Most of these men, if not all, like herself, have been neurotic,
and a neurosis in one person does not cure a neurosis in another.
They have always been the wrong men. I am sure this last man is
no exception. He sent her to me. Why? I fancy the answer lies in
his own unanalysed or inadequately analysed conflict. He wants
her, *and*, he does not want her. His instinct wants her at the
moment, but his ego or brain recognizes what I recognize, and
that is, that what she requires is to place this over-weaning
transference upon somebody who is competent to analyse her, to
reveal the conflicting elements within her fully and clearly to her
consciousness, and eventually to place her ego in charge of their
adjustment to each other and to reality. This, as her lover probably knows or senses, can be achieved only by virtue of her
getting this over-weaning transference tendency of hers attached
to somebody in the role of analyst. She is suffering from hysteria,
and needs a lot put straight before she will be well enough to
make a satisfactory adjustment to lover or husband.

Perhaps it is that she needs the parent figure, which she lacked
in childhood, to facilitate her development from infantile and
adolescent conflict to a mature, adult capacity to enjoy love, and
to fit it into the social world of reality.

The confirmation of such a theory is provided by the very next
symptom which emerged. Though she was extolling her new
found love-life, it suddenly transpired that she never really succeeded in attaining full orgastic satisfaction. A capacity for full
orgastic satisfaction has been claimed by some analysts to be the
very criterion of nervous health. It is as rare to find a psychoneurotic or person really suffering from nervous trouble, who is
completely orgastically potent, as it is to find a person who gets
full orgastic satisfaction suffering from appreciable nervous ill
health. So this lady, with all her succession of 'transferences', and

occasional episodic affairs, never achieved even physical relief.

I said to her: 'You are restless.'

She admitted it was one of her most distressing symptoms: 'I cast about everywhere and I cannot find any peace. I have to keep getting up, I cannot sit in a chair and read or study. You may think I have had many affairs, but actually by far the greater part of my life has been spent without them. In fact, somehow you have brought it to my notice already that my restlessness is due not to my having a man, but to my resisting men. Although there are always some men in the offing, some stupid enough to be wanting to marry me, I try to keep away; and I am restless.'

'And when you do have them, you are not brought to rest.' (No orgasm). I said to her: 'You do not sleep very well.'

She said: 'No, my sleep is not good, and when I do sleep I am not completely asleep. All night I am working out some phantastic problem.'

I asked her: 'Do you take sleeping pills?'

She replied, 'I either have to take a good dose every night, or else I have to go to bed half plastered with drink, I used to drink because I could not face up to things, but now I either have to drink or dope in order to get even a bit of restless sleep. Why do I drink? It's the devil, I suspect, and I'm frightened of it.'

It was time to end the interview. I am tempted to remind you once again that this interview began with a declaration of 'nothing wrong with me.' Could there be much more wrong than all this? The interview began by the patient saying she 'didn't really need analysis.' Could anybody really need analysis more than this good soul?

The compilation of the case-sheet included many more matters than I have been able to record. Amongst them I will mention just two in passing. One was that this patient's very early life was lacking in adequate parental attachment, due to the absence of parental care; I think the hereditary element, though present, was relatively not so great. It is suggested, amongst other things, by the fact that her own mother and father could not live together. This led to her being rather left out of parental care from a very early age.

The other relevant case matter is that she went through a period of infantile neurosis of appreciable severity.

Before leaving the case entirely, I am inclined to mention one point that arose immediately she presented herself for her second interview, or first analytical session. She said: 'The prospect of coming to you for analysis—though I realize now that it is necessary—has made me terribly frightened. I realize now that there is a lot that is wrong with me, a lot that I won't accept. And yet, the prospect of this analysis terrifies me.'

I asked her for her associations of thought to this terror. She said: 'I think it is that I realize that what I have got to give you is *everything*. The idea of not being allowed to hold anything back, the idea of having to give my whole self up to you is somehow a terrifying idea.'

She has never given her whole self up to anyone, not even in sexual intercourse. Her anxiety has always forced her to maintain some resistance, comparable to the resistance we saw at the initial stage of her interview. My initial object was to find what she was so frightened of, for it was the fear that caused the resistance, whether to analysis in the analytical situation, or to orgasm in the sexual situation. Was she frightened of something inside her, her sexual instinct wanting to achieve its aim (orgasm)? Or was her fear due to lack of trust in the other person, analyst or lover? Feelings of security, supported by the ego, are essential before one can be free from anxiety, able to relax and to let nature take its course, whether mental or physical. This poor 'child' had evidently never achieved this sense of security, this absence of anxiety in her relationship to parent figures, or to any of their successors. Perhaps nobody had come into her life who had merited her trust. Perhaps that had been the case in childhood— and after. She, out of some dumb hope, blindly gave it to that first (unworthy) lover, and was taught a shocking lesson.

The prospects of analytical amelioration were, I felt, very considerable, providing neither the current nor any subsequent episode of this acting-out tendency swept her away on its tide before the analytical transference was sufficiently well-established to safeguard against such symptomatic expressions of her conflict.

CHAPTER XVII

AFRAID TO MARRY

THIS case reminds us that the presenting symptom, problem, or worry may give little indication of the manifold complexes which lie beneath it, and which it serves as much to cover as to express.

He was a young man in the middle twenties sent to me because his Doctor had got tired of being pestered with obsessional questionings which obviously had their source in anxiety. He was eager to help in describing all the relevant details. He said: 'My trouble is that I just can't settle down to my job. I seem to have lost interest in everything.'

The relevance of his next remarks is worth noting: 'I am engaged to be married.' After a pause, he added, 'I just want to get away from everybody and everything. I have lost interest in getting married.'

He cast about for a while, showed some restlessness in his chair, and then blurted out: 'The fact is I am dead scared of it! Oh, yes, I have been running to my Doctor. All he can tell me is that I am in a fog.'

Presently I asked him to tell me the history of his 'illness'. He said: 'Well, I will tell you the tail end of it. We got engaged at Christmas, and we were quite happy about it. Then, as we collected things for a home, I began to see them all as shackles holding me down. I seem to have got frightened of marriage, frightened of sex. I seem to have hardly any sexual desire. The point is this. We have been excellent friends. We have had lovely holidays together, just hiking in the country. We have been doing that sort of thing for eighteen months. We have never been away from each other unless circumstances forced us to be. No, we have never had any sexual intercourse. There has never been any suggestion of such a thing from either side. We have practically kept sex out of our relationship, apart from discussing it.'

After a little hesitation, during which he was obviously battling with resistances, he said to me: 'There were two damned silly incidents: Once when we were out hiking, she teased me a lot.

She kept on teasing me, so I just caught her, and put her over my knee. After this it seemed that she often liked to tease me, and I did the same again, put her over my knee, and spanked her. Sounds silly, doesn't it? Sometimes I used to get fits of depression. I got her to take her shoes off, and beat me on the bottom with them; but it did no good. So then, I tried doing the same to her. Well, I don't know whether she liked it; anyway, she did not seem to mind very much.'

It occurs to one to reflect here that even the most unsophisticated girl commonly seems willing to endure a good many aberrations for the sake of winning her man. I do not think she is usually wise in doing so, unless, of course, she happens to be on the same immature emotional level as he is. She may win him by these devices, but it is possible that, in some cases at least, she may win someone who is not of great value to her emotionally.

He continued: 'Oh, no, as you put it, our 'intimacies' have not been confined to that. On our last holiday I used to go and say good night to her, and on two or three occasions she came in and lay on top of my bed. A few times after that she slipped into the bed with me. Neither of us had any inclination to do anything sexual. We used just to discuss the plans for the next day, and that was the end of it.'

As his conversation lagged somewhat, I felt disposed to ask him a few questions. 'You say you have known her for three years?'

'Yes.'

'All that time have you ever had any inclination to do anything sexual?'

'No. The first year that I knew her we only kissed twice, but we have been kissing during the last eighteen months. I can't be bothered with a lot of kissing.' Then a curious contradiction seemed to emerge. He said: 'I sometimes get an erection when kissing her, but I have no desire to do anything about it. We have never touched each other. We are more good friends than good lovers. I take good care of her, but the sex side doesn't go down with me. I feel I am just making an ass of myself. The chaps at work talk a lot of sex, and about girls. I don't like it. I tell them to shut up. No, I have never had any previous girl friend.'

It would seem that this particular friendship developed out of what

was simply a hiking association, and I was beginning to wonder
whether this patient might conceivably be a repressed homosexual.
So I asked him for some details of the history of his sexual development. The answers to these questions were as curious as the rest of
his story. With regard to 'alleged first sexual incident', he said:
'At the age of eleven or twelve I had a rabbit, and I thought I
had been cruel to it; I thought I ought to punish myself, so I gave
myself the torture of hanging on to a beam in the roof of the shed.
I hung on to it until I was in agony. While doing this I got an
erection and some moisture. From then on, perhaps you would
say, my emotional interest has been to make myself suffer.' (His
super-ego would make him suffer for entertaining the id-enemy.
Cruelty to the rabbit symbolizes self-castration. He is the victim
of conflict between the various structural levels of his psyche.)
'I used to tie myself up. I tried to burn myself. These experiences
produced erection, and something, though no ejaculation. I went
to see my doctor about getting engaged because I wondered if
these curious actions of mine had prejudiced me against getting
married. No, I have never masturbated. Whenever I got any
erection, I used to get frightened, and run away from the whole
idea.'

When the mature form of sexuality is frustrated or inhibited
('tied up' and 'burnt') and particularly when it is repressed, there
is a tendency for libido (the energy of the sexual instinct) to
regress—that is to say, to *go back* to an earlier stage of development—and reactivate immature component instincts. Freud
aroused a lot of opposition when he described the emotional or
'sexual' life of the child as that of a *polymorphous pervert*. But that
theory is the only one that explains the existence of such things as
sexual perversions and the tendency for frustrated libido to
regress and re-activate them. There is evidence that psychoneurotic
symptoms are not formed directly from the energy of the mature
sexual instinct but from the energy of the immature, infantile,
component instincts. If these are expressed as such, we have the
perversions; if they are repressed it is their energy, displaced by
and combined with, that of the repressing forces, that is the
dynamic power behind the symptoms of a psychoneurosis. Thus,
perversions are regarded as the *positive* expression of the *com-*

ponent instincts of sexuality, while psychoneurotic symptoms are regarded as their *negative* form.

This patient with his sexual interest in bottom-smacking and sado-masochism, showed signs of a regression of sexuality from its inhibited and repressed, genital organisation back to a more infantile, 'bottom' (or anal-sadistic) level of interest. Could anxiety be relieved sufficiently by analysis to coax it forward to a mature form? Otherwise his activities would continue to be divided between further *repressing* it, with neurotic consequences, such as anxiety, and *expressing* it as an aberration of sexuality, that is to say, as a perversion, or to continue to do what he was already doing, namely a symptomatic expression of both sides of his conflict.

Generally speaking, the tendency to repress component-instincts or potential perversions is stronger than the tendency to repress the mature form of sexuality. The latter can be made to fit into the social-religious structure; it can be accepted by society, the super-ego and the ego, whereas the former is usually unacceptable. Thus, regression of libido, when mature forms of sexuality are inhibited and repressed, does not lead to a solution of the problem, but rather to a still more powerful repression of the reactivated component instincts, or to an intensification of the conflict.

The patient proceeded with his story: 'I often envied girls, I envied them their neatness and their tidiness. I have often wished I were a girl. I wanted to wear a kilt as a compromise.'

'When was puberty?'

'I suppose about fifteen or sixteen; that was when I had my first wet dream. It happened very rarely, only about once in three or four months.'

It is not exceptional in one's clinical experience to find that sex-repressed patients manage to extend their sex repression to their physiological functions; I would say even beyond their sexual physiology. The forces of repression seem powerful enough not only to create scotomata, or blind spots in the mind, but also some functional arrest in the body itself. This shows us how powerful mental forces, such as those of repression, can be in their effects.

It transpired that this young man had been engaged for six months, and increasingly worried over the engagement for the past four or five months. He said: 'I have always been worried. I am the worrying sort, but never have I been so worried as this. It came to a head a couple of months ago, and since then I seem to have been in a sort of fog.' He added: 'I'm not interested in sex.'

When I asked him if his fiancee was interested, he replied: 'I don't know; I think quite probably, but it's only a guess.' He said: 'Sex has never troubled me at all.' Then he added: 'Except for that trying-to-make-myself-suffer business, if you can call that sex. That did give me a little worry, but my worry came to a head with this engagement.'

Becoming more confidential, presently he said to me: 'Do you know, Doctor, what I should really like to do, what is my real ambition?' I did not know. He said: 'I would like to go on a long exploration. I would like to lead, or to be a member of, an expedition to the North Pole. (!) I like the idea of cold climates and hardship. I would be in the seventh heaven if I were going on such an expedition instead of having to face up to this marriage idea.'

It may not impress the unanalysed when I draw attention to the symbolical significance of the frozen North as a symbol of a-sexuality—as far removed from the flames of passion as possible. Incidentally, this is psychologically related to this young man's only 'sexual' pleasure, being in the form of what might normally be regarded as the antithesis of sexuality, namely pain or suffering. It is as though his super-ego would permit him to enjoy only punishment, punishment for the sexuality which he has repressed, punishment for sexuality *in spite of* his having repressed it. It will probably not be appreciated when I say that he had repressed it on account of 'castration anxiety'. This is related to pain or punishment becoming *by association* the crime, namely sexuality, for which the punishment takes place.

But all these things are as deep in this patient's unconscious as they are in that of the unanalysed reader, and a first interview is the most inappropriate time to make any interpretation. When he proceeded to tell me a few anxiety and obsessional symptoms, I was in no way surprised. We can hardly get such a massive repression without some leakage of the repressed emotions in the form of symptoms. He said: 'Yes, I have got into a state since this engagement. I have been going round checking the taps all over the old house, and then going back and checking them all over again. Another thing that has worried me, and kept me awake at nights—Doctor, I'm afraid you will think me mad—since my girl friend slipped into my bed, although nothing happened, we didn't even kiss . . . yet I am tormented ever since with anxiety that she is going to have a baby.'

This remark of his reminds me of a young woman patient whom I once saw, who was afraid that if a man passed along the pavement on the opposite side of the street, she, my patient, would become pregnant! Such symptoms serve to bring it home to us how powerful may be the repressed instincts, and how strong their tendency, emanating from their undischarged energy, to influence our thoughts, even in opposition to our reason. A little more and they can sweep away reason, in which case we have delusions and psychoses.

I am rather ashamed to say that at the end of this interview (as recorded) with this young man, I telephoned his doctor, and said that whatever he, the doctor, thought, I myself had very little hope that I would ever be able to make his patient well enough to be happily married, particularly as the young man could only attend about once a week. The doctor said: 'Well, I don't know what else we can do with him, so you had better have a try!' However, we agreed that there was no point at the moment in his braving the marriage, as it was an absolute certainty that he was miles away from even the beginning of potency.

My conception is that there are various degrees of impotence, measureable by the distance (sexually) between the man and the woman. This man had never been conscious even of the phantasy of intercourse. He had indeed a very long path to travel, perhaps over the North Pole, and back again! He was more concerned to turn off the taps of sexuality than to run the risk of their slightest leakage—and yet he was awake at nights wondering whether the worst had inadvertently happened, and 'castration', in the form of his fiancee's pregnancy, would overtake him. I could not tell how much analysis would be required before he would show the first sign of being able to face that enormous repressed castration phantasy.

To my discredit, this was a case about which I proved to be

mistaken. He was one of my keenest analysands, though keenness does not always ensure success. When he heard that I was reluctant to treat him, he moved heaven and earth to persuade or force me to do so. His very potency in this respect initiated the first revision of my estimate of him. Indeed, it is the fact that nobody would now recognize in him the person of the first interview, which makes it possible for me to publish the substance of it.

CHAPTER XVIII

THE STRONG MAN

THE popular conception of a psychoneurotic man is possibly that of some rather contemptible, effeminate and garrulous individual, full of childish anxieties and hypochondriacal symptoms.

The following case may help to show that this is by no means always the case. This patient, like a good many other psychoneurotics, was the absolute antithesis of this popular idea. He arrived obviously full of reluctances and resistances. Practically everything he said was an under-statement, the degree of which emerged only in the fullness of time. Therefore, it is not very easy to do justice to him at his first interview.

I was confronted by a big strong, manly and athletic-looking person in the late thirties. He regarded me silently and grimly. After the usual mundane questions, the answers to which happened to reveal that he was the son of a North Irish clergyman, and that he had been educated at Belfast University, I asked him what brought him to see me. He was evidently in no hurry to unburden himself. What I wish to point out here is that the reasons for coming, or even the complaints, first detailed by almost any patient often amount merely to derivatives acting as a mask for what is really wrong. Not that the patient *wants* to mask it. Owing to the forces of repression it has been masked in this way from himself, and substituted by these derivatives. *He* is taken-in by them, but we need not be.

The first thing he told me, in answer to my question as to what brought him to see me, was that it was due to trouble with his wife. Evidently, she, for some inadequate reason, wished to be freed from her marriage to him. At first he was inclined, rather half-heartedly, to blame the war, and the months of separation occasioned by his service abroad. Amongst the truths that emerged subsequently, indicative of how much lay beneath this first mild statement, was the fact that when he gave expression to his thoughts and feelings in the presence of his wife, such a storm of emotional energy burst forth, almost shaking the rafters of their home, that the rather limited young woman was terrified out of her wits—although he had no intention whatsoever of terrifying her—and her one over-riding impulse was to run away from him.

When I asked him if this marital trouble was all that was wrong, he admitted to 'a little restlessness', and added, 'It has made me take certain actions'. This again was a gross understatement. It would hardly be an exaggeration to say that this man could not sit still for five minutes. He was at sixes and sevens with himself and with everything, in an intolerable state of tension, which, in spite of iron control, periodically burst out like a volcanic eruption. The 'certain actions', to which he referred so mildly and vaguely, included flaming rows with some of his senior officers, and a passionate love affair, or sex affair, with a woman he had met abroad. This affair he had only half attempted to conceal from his wife; it was the excuse for, rather than the real cause of, her urgent insistence to be free.

A third matter to which he mildly referred, also proved to be very near the crux of his overwhelming trouble. He said: 'I had a very stormy family life when I was a boy, and underlying everything that has happened to me since, has been this feeling of wanting to be completely independent of my family, as far away from them as possible.' He added: 'Now I am wondering whether I was really justified in being so determined to get away.'

All this meant, first, that he had laboured under a conviction that his trouble was his family, and so, if only he could get away from them and that atmosphere, he would be perfectly all right; and, second, that, having got away from them all, he found he was just as restless and impossible without them, though still reluctant to face up to the fact that the trouble lay within himself, his own disposition, temperament, and character.

This was a case in which one had to be very careful, quiet, silent and receptive. Any attempt at interpretation, for instance a hint at the truth of what I have just written, would possibly have precipitated one of those flaming rows which I subsequently learnt about; or, if it had not precipitated a row, it would have aroused emotions in him the control of which would have increased his tension, and made him want to keep away from me. Such a mistake would have been a pity, as this was a man who not only required help very badly, but who would easily be disposed to reject the help he required in the same way as he had rejected his parents and family.

These things were, of course, not stated at this first interview, but they were intuitively sensed. I could feel that it would be a strain for me successfully to handle this difficult individual—difficult because so rigid, sensitive and individualistic. It was easy to conclude that all persons with whom he had come in contact had probably felt this strain, and, sooner or later, avoided him, as his wife was striving to do. It is natural to try to avoid situations of strain, or persons whose qualities are such that they impose psychological inhibitions upon our own freedom, and thereby force us to endure our tensions unrelieved. The psychologist can only help such persons if he is able himself to tolerate a good deal of frustration and strain. Anyhow, in his case there is the clock which limits the period of his endurance. I could say, however, that no strain which I might be called upon to bear would be comparable to the tension which this unfortunate man had to put up with, from intrapsychic causes, irrespective of the company he was in.

As frequently happens in such cases, he had tossed about from one place to another, more or less all round the world, fruitlessly trying to gain some relief. Perhaps it is an idea common to us all, that the only thing we need do is to find the right environment, and our stresses and strains will be at an end, and everything will be satisfactory. In other words, we all endeavour to manipulate reality to suit us, as though that were the only 'therapy' which we could imagine. If nature has been kind to us we may not be entirely wrong. Those unfortunate people with internal and unconscious sources of tension, comparable to that of this patient, naturally, unconsciously or consciously, try to find their own remedies in the accepted manner. They never find them. Even if they go from one end of the earth to the other, they never find relief, for the source of their intolerable tension is within them. It emanates from their own repressed complexes, and unless these are brought to consciousness and dealt with, they continue to be the victims of 'insoluble' conflict.

Those who, in desperation, rush to the bottle or to drugs are similarly constituted. One of the nicest men I have ever met, a doctor, who was a drug addict, said to me: 'Before I took to drugs, the *feelings* within me were indescribably intolerable. Without apparent cause, no matter where I was, or whatever the circumstances, I was sort-of 'boiling' inside with feelings of indescribable agony in my mind. Half the time I was struggling against suicide. Something *had* to be done to relieve my condition. I just could not bear it. Nobody could have put up with it. It is worse than acute pain. It is a sort of mixture of boiling, itching, scratching. You want to claw at yourself, scratch your brain, but you can't. Nobody who has not had these feelings can understand the relentless strain it is to endure them; and, on top of that, to put a bland, civilized face towards the world, (a pretence of normality, a 'friend of everyone'!) makes it still more impossible to endure. You asked me why I started the drugs? Well, perhaps, you will begin to understand from what I have said. I did not want to commit suicide because that would be so heart-breaking for my family, and it is a very final and irrevocable thing, isn't it? One likes to think or to hope that 'while there is life, there is hope.' Taking a drug to lessen the agony (which it does at first) is a compromise —a compromise between suicide, and the wish to live free from this agony. The trouble about drug-taking, especially morphia, is that it is a run-away horse. You start with quarter of a grain; within a week it's no good, and you have to increase it to a half, and before you know where you are, you are in the major doses, taking enough to kill a dozen men a day, and going rapidly downhill, physically as well as mentally.'

Can such agony as this drug-addict described to me be purely psychogenic? The answer is, it can be, and it is. The patient, whose first interview I have been describing, had, surprising to relate, not taken to drugs, nor even to drink; there was something in his mental constitution that steeled him against giving way to such a weakness. It was something, which, at the same time, demanded perfections of him, always beyond what were humanly possible. Most of the time he endured his internal agonies more successfully than other people endured them. Occasionally he broke out with some more or less violent mode of relief. Fortunately his violent outbursts were confined to talking, or rather to shouting. There was something in his character which effectively inhibited any physical expression of violence, something which is, perhaps, lacking in the wife-beater, delinquent, and criminal; but this did not make his inward psychological state any more comfortable *for him*.

What had perhaps brought his condition home to him more convincingly than any previous episode in his life was the fact that his wife, whom he had always thought was 'on his side', was now openly revealing her determination to be rid of him. Subsequently I gained the impression that what his wife found so difficult to endure was chiefly the rigid strength of his *character*. She had said that she wanted freedom 'to develop her own personality'. In his presence there was room for only one personality—his!—though he may have been right in his contention that what she really wanted was, 'like all women', to wear the trousers herself; and this he could not even pretend to allow.

Presently, I had to insist upon his telling me rather more clearly what was the purpose of his coming to see me. He said: 'One has had a lot of stresses and strains . . . and that has made this restlessness worse. . . . I really wanted to chat with somebody who was outside the whole thing. You will have to get a clearer picture of it than I have myself.'

I asked: 'A clearer picture of what?'

He replied: 'The present situation. I know I will have to find some employment. Perhaps I will have to re-cast my ideas. I feel that I am faced with a very difficult problem. I am wondering what is the best thing to do. First, I suppose, one has to find some regular occupation, so that one is occupied. I am finding it hard to decide what is the best step to take. Perhaps for the first time in my life I find it impossible to make a decision.'

It is such vague complaints as these at a first interview which commonly mean a great deal more than the dramatic symptoms of hysteria and anxiety states. These remarks were really amongst the most blatant under-statements which he had made to me. He talked of finding employment, something to keep him occupied. Now the truth is that this man was, at that time, totally unfit, on account of his state of nervous illness, for any employment whatsoever. 'Something to keep me occupied!' This man was occupied day and night with the most acute and intolerable conflict imaginable, and none the less severe because it was nearly all at an unconscious level. There was only one appropriate 'decision' for him to make, one which I feared he might resist, even, as it were, to his dying breath, and that decision was to be treated by regular daily analysis.

I wondered whether it might prove a little tactless to say this to him at this point. Had he consulted a hospital psychiatrist, rather than an analyst, and had the psychiatrist appreciated the unexpressed agony in the man's mind, it is conceivable that he might have recommended his admission to a hospital for nervous trouble. But I felt sure that in this man's case, such a recommendation would have proved inappropriate. I tried to draw him out a little more.

He told me of a succession of troubles (I am sure they were all of a psychogenic nature) which had overtaken him during his many years of war service, especially in the later years. From difficulties or impossibilities in his personal contacts, they had progressed to such familiar things as suspected gastric ulcer, dysentery and skin diseases, some of them requiring hospital attention.

It then transpired that this particularly virile-looking man had had no sexual relationship for something like six months or more. He explained this fact in the following way: 'The last time I had intercourse with my wife, she broke down at the end of it. I saw that she was struggling with her tears, and then she broke down, and wept and wept. I could see that it was having a bad effect upon her.'

I, stupidly, said, "Why?"

He replied: 'I suppose there was something different about it to what it had been previously.'

My private reflection upon this bit of news was that his wife sensed herself married to a very sick man, mentally or nervously sick. To her mind that sickness had expressed itself in what seemed *to her* the worst possible way, namely by infidelity. (She was repressing her reactive hate, but she thereby felt unconsciously that she was accepting 'destruction'). In these circumstances submitting to intercourse had been a great strain upon her, and very difficult to endure. Fortunately he had not pressed this imposition upon her again.

Finally, looking at his tense, strong, ugly, masculine face, I ventured to remark: 'The "stresses and strains" have not become less. You can't come to a "decision" because you are all bottled-up. The fact is that you are ill at present.'

Somewhat to my surprise, this great he-man suddenly broke down; he burst into tears, and sobbed like a child. I left the room, and returned ten minutes later, merely to give him an appointment for the next day.

The psychopathology of this case might well fill many chapters, but as the principal study in this book is that of first interviews, and how to conduct them, I shall resist the temptation to embark upon a lengthy explanation. Another reason for not going further with the matter is that details of family history and upbringing, all of which were relevant to his condition, might incur some little risk of revealing his identity, particularly as he has now become a well-known personality.

However, in justice to him, perhaps I should add that increasing insight into his own condition, coupled with recovery, has so increased his, now remarkable, insight into people and their follies, that he might be excused a certain feeling of 'superiority' over the average run of mankind. His remaining 'fault', if any, is his completely uncompromising attitude towards the hypocracies and meannesses of man. Some might not care for his ruthless exposure of human stupidities, frailties, and meannesses, but, knowing him, one gets to like his unvarying truthfulness and even perhaps his contempt for the weaknesses which he himself is incapable of stooping to—or tolerating.

Indeed his previous illness can now be seen in a new light. It can be seen that he was ill because he had a dynamic energy within him—bottled up within him—that must tear the *inside*, if it cannot find a permissible, conflict-free outlet. It has been shown that, released from repression, this energy is the harbinger of *health* (instead of illness), nervous and mental health, greater than that which is average or normal. In the light of what has transpired it may prove to be even the power-component of genius. The dynamic ingredients of genius if kept under a repressive cloak will cause more illness, than will those of a mummy similarly confined! The 'heart once pregnant with celestial fire' may burn itself up if it cannot dissipate its heat and energy; and the 'Cromwell, guiltless of his country's blood' may become 'guilty' of internal self-destruction.

CHAPTER XIX

HATE BEFORE LOVE

IT is a curious fact that although the things which a patient relates to one at a first interview are always a clue to the nature of his trouble, and most relevant to the essence of his illness, they are, at the same time, a seemingly deliberate, misleading paraphrase of it.

For instance, in the following case, the man's illness was one which took all his attention and emotional energy *away from* normal sexual-social adjustments. He proved to be far too strongly preoccupied with what amounted to the dramatization of an aggressive complex, to have any emotional energy left over for love or sexual relationship; and yet the very first thing he said to me was: 'I am very much in love with a girl.'

Perhaps the explanation of this is that the individual is trying to adjust to what he and others regard as a normal, understandable form of interest and activity. It is not *his* individual, personal form at all, at least not while he has his illness, and it is this attempt at normal adjustment (abnormal for him) which brings the psychopathology of his mental-emotional pattern to a head. So long as we walk about on land and breathe air, we are alive and well, but if the idea were instilled into our mind that we *ought to be* fishes, and we tried to live in the sea, we would find that there was a great deal wrong! This man presumably did not fully realize how ill he was until he found that he was, or rather *ought to be*, 'very much in love with a girl.'

He added: 'That is the reason why I have come to see you.' I remained silent, assuming that if that was all there was to it, he would certainly not have come to see me. Presently he added, 'I think she is on the point of accepting me.' The mystery deepened. Finally, he added the real clue: 'What I am afraid of is that I may fall out of love with her at any time.' I guessed that he had very good reasons for his fear, and, presently, some of them emerged. He said: 'It's happened before with other girls. I can chase a girl all right, and I seem determined to win her. I work like anything, getting rid of all the obstacles and any reluctance. She *has* to accept me. I think I must be a most determined wooer. I may say that I have always been a fighter. I fight like mad to get my way in everything. And I succeed. I get the girl. I always win. The tragedy is that, however quickly she is won, however swiftly I pursued her and caught her, once she accepts me, once she stops running away, once she agrees to marry me, it is as though I stop chasing her, and race for my life in the opposite direction! Once they accept me, I always want to get away. To tell you the truth, it has happened only recently, and here I can see it coming again.' He continued: 'I have studied a bit of psychology, and I think it is tied up with what you people call a mother-fixation, but, in my case, the mother-fixation is not a love-fixation, it is a *hate*-fixation.'

Nothing this patient said ever proved more correct than this statement of his. It transpired that he had been brought up, practically from birth, by a stepmother who outclassed in harshness and severity all the stepmothers of all the harrowing legends. In due course this appeared to be most relevant to the patient's psychopathology, which went much deeper than that of the current problem with which he opened. In fact, it penetrated so deeply into his nature that one wondered sometimes whether any stepmother, however harsh and tyrannical, could possibly be wholly responsible for the result. One felt it would take more than one individual lifetime to produce a compulsive pattern as all-powerful as his proved to be.

He went on to tell me some details of his life history. He said: 'There were six of us. I was the youngest. My mother died shortly after my birth. The maternity nurse stayed on to look after us, and before long she married my widowed father. I cannot tell you the intensity of the atmosphere of *fear* in which we were brought up. My father was too busy to know what was going on. That stepmother was *the* most subtle criminal that ever lived. One of her clever tricks was to put each child against the others, so as to ensure that we never combined against her. Perhaps my sister, the eldest of the family, had the worst time. She used to be thrashed every day, and made to do all the work. At fifteen she ran away from home, but was brought back and thrashed. She ran away again six months later, but again without success. When she inherited quite a sum of money that my mother had left her, the stepmother changed her tactics for the time being, and managed to spend the lot of it on herself. However, all that was nothing. It was the treatment which *I* received that affected me most, and I was the youngest.

'Now, why is it, Doctor, although I can abuse my stepmother like this to you, I cannot bear anyone else to say anything against her. I still support her. She has money each week out of my earnings. What do you make of that? When I had a nervous breakdown fifteen years ago, the psychotherapist who was treating me eventually said to me: 'You will never be well until you have nothing more to do with your stepmother. Cast her out.' Well, I didn't cast her out, but I felt so furious with him for suggesting such a thing that I cast him out. I refused to see him again."

Perhaps this is an example of the inadvisability of trying to 'cure' a patient, or even to influence him, by advice, correction, or merely by interpretation (except of resistances), *until* his transference to you is fully established. This patient's 'transference' was still attached to his wicked old stepmother, the alleged cause of all his troubles, and when the hospital psychotherapist joined combat with the power she exercised over the patient's mind, however unconsciously, the psychotherapist was vanquished immediately, no matter how sound his advice. That was an error of technique.

At an interview the story does not usually emerge chronologically. The following gradually transpired: the patient went to a boarding school at fourteen: 'I was there introduced to masturbation, and have struggled against it ever since, for twenty-five years. I had a strong guilt complex about sex, but that is better now. I may tell you that since meeting this girl, six months ago, I have not even *wanted* to masturbate. I don't think that has been entirely due to the idea that I would not be potent or able to satisfy her sexually, if I didn't stop it, because there has not even been the want.

'I have been to two other psychiatrists before, chiefly on account of sleeplessness. Immediately after the war it was assumed that my illness was due to war-shock, and I went through some so-called abreaction treatment in a hospital. Doctor, it is something far deeper than anything that happened in the war. I myself found

that out in the course of the treatment. I am faced with the consequences, tragedy if you will, of my present position with this
girl. I have come here to have the whole matter cleared up. I
am sure it goes right back to my infancy.

'Up to the age of seven, I suffered from bed-wetting. I was
beaten by my stepmother practically every morning from the age
of three or four for it. One of her tricks was to get a sister of mine
to go up to my bedroom to feel if my bed was wet, and to report
to her. Of course, the girl was too terrified of her to give a false
report. I tried all sorts of deceptions to conceal it, but my sister
would always discover it, and report. Then I would lie in bed
trembling with terror, and waiting for the inevitable beating.
People have no idea what a terrible thing a beating can be to a
child, physically as well as mentally. They have repressed it. I
remember everything. The pain apart from the terror is unendurable.'

An interesting addendum to this little story, and, at the same
time, an interesting confirmation of a developing transference in
this patient is the following: One day, a few months later, when
I went to collect him from the waiting-room, he was sitting bolt
upright in his chair, literally sweating with anxiety. He spoke
not a word until I had him lying on the settee, and then, after a
silence, he said: 'I heard your footsteps in the hall, approaching
the waiting-room, and I could almost have sworn that I heard
you make some sound outside, like the rattling of sticks. It was
exactly the same as I felt when I was an infant, waiting for the stepmother to come into my bedroom, and lay about me with the stick.
I can remember now that from the moment my sister would leave
my room, having discovered that I had wet the bed again as
usual, I would sit there in a state of terror, acutely alive to every
movement and every sound in the house. Finally, after what
seemed like an agony of suspense (I know exactly what a man
feels like in the condemned cell), I would hear her footstep in the
hall below—like I heard yours. I would hear the rattle of sticks
in the hall-stand as she selected one, and then every step up the
staircase to my bedroom. It was a nightmare. But it was worse
than a nightmare, for there was no happy awakening. No matter
how much I begged for mercy, and screamed and cried, the flog-
ging would be executed to the last blow. Then she would walk

out with some such snarling remark as, "That'll teach you!"
Evidently, a few minutes ago, I was expecting the same treatment from you!'

It transpired that not the least of this patient's symptom-pro-
duced problems was that connected with the management of his
large store, of which he was in charge. One might assume that
having been the victim of such savage treatment throughout his
childhood and adolescence, he would have some sympathy for other
people, and that the last thing he would tend towards would be
tyranny over them. This assumption proved to be incorrect,
though in a way not entirely so. I cannot describe how completely
his very abundant and vigorous emotional energy was absorbed
in a relationship to his employees comparable only to that of his
stepmother towards himself and the other children. Even his
phantasies were almost exclusively of this nature. He would
imagine himself going to the shop, and, as he said to me in the
identical, snarling tone of voice which his stepmother used, 'Sack-
ing the lot!' He imagined himself grinding out, with the utmost
harshness to men and women individually: 'There's your hat!
OUT!'

Indeed, the compulsion of this sort of behaviour had, up to the
time of his analysis, commonly over-ridden his common sense and
control. He told me that before coming, he had actually sacked
not less than eight assistants in six months! The sackings had
been passionately emotional, hate affairs. He was very prone to a
paranoid illusion that people were combining together to get an
advantage over him. In his phantasy they were villains, and no
treatment could be too bad for them ('Sack the lot!'). Had he been
able to do so, he would probably have murdered the lot! But,
nevertheless, he was sane enough to suspect that it was all due to
something pathological in himself.

There was, however, another side to his phantasy. It was the
opposite. If the villains, or the particular villain of the moment,
did not react to his aggression with aggression, but, on the contrary, with humility, self-abasement, or distress, then our tyrant
would become the soul of pity. He would be overwhelmed with
kindness, and compelled to become the saviour and benefactor
instead of the destroyer.

All this led to some very interesting and even amusing episodes.

For instance, at one time he repeatedly told me of a selfish brute of a man who sat, occupying more than a fair-share of his seat, in the tube train in which he travelled to work. This great brute spread his elbows over both adjacent seat-arms to hold the newspaper he was reading, and thus gave the persons sitting immediaately beside him a very poor deal. For a time my patient was obsessed with a phantasy in which this man figured as the great ogre or bully. He imagined himself, presumably in the role of 'Jack the Giant Killer', tearing this man to pieces, destroying him in a sort of sadistic murder. The point was that he was destroying something intolerably bad. These phantasies he would modify, in accordance with his sense of reality, into such ideas as challenging the man to come outside and fight it out, and so on.

Eventually, one day, to bring the matter to a head, he took his courage in both hands, and deliberately sat next to the great bully. Presently, having steeled himself to anticipating a combat comparable to that of St. George and the Dragon, and, with great control, modifying his approach to something within rational limits, he said to the man: 'Do you mind very much if I have a portion of the arm of my seat?' Instead of replying with the expected slap in the face, immediately the great ogre tucked both his elbows into himself, folded up his newspaper, apologized most profusely, and became very affable. My patient's phantasy crumbled in the dust. He felt disposed to reassure the old gentleman, and to persuade him to put his elbow on the arm again.

However, matters were not so simple in the store, and, delay as he might, the result was an all too frequent series of dismissals, and engagings of new staff. As analysis progressed, the psychopathology of this condition revealed itself as follows: The intense hatred of his stepmother, generated in infancy, and constantly stimulated by her aggression, was naturally repressed through his fear of her. It had become the chief emotional ingredient of his repressed unconscious. Practically all his capacity for hatred and aggression had gone into this complex. Overlaying this he had built up a reaction-formation, and in consequence he was superficially one of the most normal and affable, if not self-abasing, of men. But this was only at the expense of holding in a raging furnace of repressed hatred. The pressure of this hatred was too great to be consistently held in or controlled. His ego would be

E

busy looking for opportunities to relieve himself of some modicum of it. This predisposed him to illusions or delusions that there were villains or a villain about, meriting his destructive aggression. (It is interesting to see here how a super-ego is formed in the image of the parent-figure.)

Occasionally, some employee, actually one employee after another, would be assigned to the appropriate role in the phantasy, tormented, and eventually sacked, or chased away in terror from his employment. Of course, there was another side to the complex. Whereas villains (displacements of the hated stepmother) had to be destroyed, poor little helpless things like the victim-children had to be saved and succoured. If anybody were sufficiently un-aggressive or humble to fit this latter role, my patient would be his or her champion.

Unfortunately, for people with this paranoid type of phantasy, it is a fact that though it starts with an illusion of hostility on the part of the other person (through projection of their own repressed hostility) the expression of it commonly and naturally arouses reactive hostility in the other party, and so tends to confirm and to make real that which originally was an illusion.

I imagine that it was through some such process as this that Hitler, fearing the 'encirclement of Germany' by enemies, eventually succeeded in making his phantasy a very real reality.

The analysis of this patient was not completed until his transference, the first stage of which has been seen, had so developed that the analyst was assigned the leading role in his phantasy, and the interpretation and dissolution of it was worked out during the actual analytical sessions. However, it never became so intense as one anticipated, for it is technically correct to interpret transference, particularly negative transference, soon after it arises, (even if it is not visible), provided it has established itself sufficiently, and received sufficient expression, indirect or direct, for its interpretation to be credible to the patient.

In view of the almost complete absorption of this patient's emotional energy in his hate-complex, whether in expressing it, or in the strain and stress of holding it back from expression, there is small wonder that not much of his emotional potentialities were left over for a heterosexual love life. In view of his chief and almost exclusive pre-occupation with these hate-emotions, his relationship to a girl-friend or a wife seemed almost beside the point. Emotionally he was elsewhere engaged. Thus, he had every reason to feel concern or anxiety at the situation he had inadvertently got himself into: 'very much in love with a girl.'

How could he be very much in love with a girl, or sufficiently in love with her to maintain a love interest adequate to satisfy her requirements, if he were, day and night, fighting ogres, derivatives of the erstwhile stepmother, (or, in so far as he was on the stepmother's side [super-ego], derivatives of her enemies), and fighting them as though his very life depended upon the outcome of the battle? Only when this complex of his had been made fully conscious, and worked out, was he emotionally free to deal with his business rationally, and his love-life emotionally.

This excerpt may indicate to the reader that, like this patient, personal relationships in all of us, whether at first interviews or otherwise, are always influenced, however unwittingly, by our irrevelant complexes or emotional patterns, inherited and acquired.

CHAPTER XX

INVOLUNTARY RELIEF OF TENSION

THE dynamic energy of the mind, generated by the body's metabolic processes, can express itself in a variety of ways. The basic channels of expression are naturally the inherited ones, called instincts. Subsequent to birth, the baby, infant, or small child, impressionable and malleable in comparison to the adult, acquires certain patterns of emotional expression based upon the inherited ones (instincts), and amounting to minor modifications and elaborations of these. (In my opinion—not an orthodox one—this is a process of the formation, sometimes Lamarckian-wise, of something equivalent to new 'instincts'—in process of formation.)

But, what I am concerned with in this chapter is that the various expressions of the dynamic energy of the mind include not only instinctual ones, but also all the various forms, modifications and elaborations, morbid and otherwise, which these inherited patterns have acquired in the malleable years of early life. Together these reaction patterns, inherited and acquired, promote not only our survival, individual and racial, but also the development of the body social.

If an individual is blessed or cursed with an undue quantity of this basic dynamic energy, he may have difficulty in relieving it along the prescribed, customary channels, to the optimum level consistent with nervous, mental, and physical—and social—well-being. Thus, we get aberrations from the normal, both in the direction of creditable activity, even genius, and in the direction of abnormalities, such as nervous, mental or physical ill-health, deflection, and delinquency. More often than is popularly supposed the individual is not himself the arbiter of what particular direction his mental energy may take.

The case, the first interview of which I am going to describe, is one in which some of this, perhaps excessive, dynamic energy, took an unusual or deviated course during infancy. Incidentally, a bit of this sort of thing can be discovered during the analysis of almost all nervously and mentally ill people—to which categories we all more or less belong, whether we know it or not. In this case we have evidence of the deviated direction of emotional energy as early as four years of age, evidence which suggests that it started at some inaccessible period much earlier. There are very definite signs of its full establishment as early as six and a half or seven.

The patient was a middle-aged woman, married, and with a grown-up family. She was blunt, forceful, and a bit jerky in her expression of herself. She gave me the impression that she was covering up a nice kindly disposition under a cloak of slightly aggressive brusqueness. At first she just sat and stared at me in a non-commital way that might have been erroneously interpreted as slight hostility. She waited for me to ask the usual mundane questions.

When, after recording her answers to these, I asked her what she complained of, she replied, with some under-statement: 'I have been struggling against nervous tension.' It transpired that what she meant by this was that she was constantly throughout her waking hours in a most uncomfortable state of anxiety or tension, which, amongst other things, caused her to maintain a tautness of practically all her bodily muscles, particularly those of her abdomen. She was very conscious of this uncomfortable condition physically and mentally. It appears that it had been present, in some degree, all through her life including childhood, but of recent years it had been mounting to an intensity which was becoming unendurable.

Presently, she added: 'And I am hypochondriacal and nervous about my health. It is absolutely idiotic!'

'Can you tell me what is your hypochondriacal fear?'

She replied with one word: 'Cancer.' She added: 'I have a fear of cancer. If I have any pain anywhere, I think it's cancer, and my fear mounts up to a panic.'

I then asked the duration of these symptoms, and she said: 'I have been a neurotic person all my life, worse for the last two or three years.'

'Have you any idea of when or how it started?'

She replied bluntly, concealing the resistance she had to overcome, and the effort it cost her: 'At the age of six I started to masturbate, and I have done it ever since.'

Later it transpired there were signs of this 'masturbation' as early as four years of age.

'Would you care to tell me what this "masturbation" is?'

'Well, I have a ridiculous childish phantasy, sometimes I encourage it on purpose, to try and relieve my tension—it does relieve it a bit temporarily—but sometimes it comes quite involuntarily, even when I least want it, and when I try to stop it, for instance, at a business meeting or something like that. It started when I was very small, and it is still the same phantasy. The phantasy is that a child is being punished; but there are some curious features which are absolutely essential. One is that the child is being punished by somebody who loves it, and the other is that the child has to feel that it is guilty and to acquiesce in the punishment. At that point I get an orgasm, involuntary, whether I want it or not.' Presently she added: 'I have never had any pleasure from sexual intercourse because of this thing.'

This patient insisted upon calling her habit 'masturbation', although that is a misnomer as there was no manual or other manipulation, indeed, her symptom amounted to a purely and exclusively mental stimulation, sometimes voluntary, sometimes involuntary. Any physical intrusion, such as that of intercourse, produced absolute frigidity. She herself took it for granted that her symptom of frigidity was the direct consequence of her sexual energy having taken this divergent or deflected course. Here she was fairly correct in her theory. Most cases of impotence and frigidity are due to some alternative practice, commonly masturbation, having gained, perhaps through excess, complete monopoly of the orgasm-producing sexual pattern. In these cases it is as though the urgency for relief of tension was too great to await social-sexual adjustment. Tension had to be relieved, and the mind, or, in some cases, we may say the body, even without the mind, found a path for relief. In minor instances of this we may have to blame our social order that puts such large obstacles in the way of normal adjustment; but in other cases, such as this one, the aetiological factors go deeper, and the aberrant pattern of tension-relief becomes so ingrained, as it were, by the energy so repetitively using the path which it has found, that it is difficult to divert it afterwards to any other channel, such as that of normal sexuality. Owing partly at least to our social order, there is an element of this sort of thing in practically every so-called normal person. Normally it is not a large enough element to exclude a varying degree of normal social-sexual adjustment, though, I believe that it detracts more or less from full orgastic potency, and so promotes a tendency to nervous ill-health—not to mention social disorders such as divorce. If the would-be reformer devoted his energies to removing the obstacles to normal development, instead of to increasing them, there would be less nervous, mental and social ills.

This patient's tension, though physiologically relieved to a certain extent, voluntarily or, if resisted, involuntarily, did not achieve an equivalent mental or psychological relief; rather the contrary, for the more her reflexes automatically discharged the intolerable tension that accumulated within her, the more they aroused worry and conflict in her mind, and these latter stimulated complexes that seemed to produce their own tension. I think, however, that there must be some basic ingredient of tension arising, not *from* her displaced or 'masturbatory' activities, but from their relative absence, due to her resistance to them, and her almost constant endeavour to inhibit them and to keep them in check. It was only when tension developed to an intolerable degree that she permitted its release, or if she did not permit it, if she still resisted, it would become too intense to be held, even with the exertion of all her powers of resistance, and it would then relieve itself automatically, as it were without her permission, and against her will.

Naturally, being the victim of such an automatic process, comparable, shall we suggest, to incontinence, she was in a state of mental worry and distress. Her attempts to put a brave face on things, and to *appear* normal, even to her husband, even during sexual intercourse, amounted to her enduring a further tension-producing effort heaped upon a load which was already too great for her to carry.

She said: 'My husband and I have had a happy married life purely because I have never divulged that I experience no sexual pleasure. His intercourse with me has always increased my feeling of tension, never relieved it, and never given me any pleasure. I have only this "private sexual intercourse" to relieve my tension. I knew in advance that when I married I would be frigid, but in spite of that I think I have made a good job of it. It is a terrible ordeal for me to have to tell anybody all this stuff. I cannot show what I feel privately. All my life I have been taught never to show my feelings.'

This was a woman of energy and initiative. As early as twenty years of age she had sought out what was perhaps recognized at that time to be the greatest authority in England, had managed, without her mother or anybody knowing it, to arrange an interview with him, and had told him what she was now telling me. She said: 'I told him I was "masturbating" day and night, and I asked him if I should marry. All he said to me was that he could not tell me. Anyhow my life has been happier since I married, though, so far as my husband is concerned, my sexuality has been just pretence. The "masturbation" has continued, but in later years not to the same extent.'

Analyst: 'Have you, perhaps, been trying to stop it?'

Patient: 'I have not the strength to stop it. I do not think I have the strength to struggle against it. It is too long established.' She then went on to a recital of her other symptoms. This I regarded as a digression, as my interest was, of course, focused upon the aetiology, origin, and development of the 'masturbation' phantasy. But this being merely an interview, I 'respected' her defences, and allowed her to continue with this digression of hers, taking the opportunity to record it as case-sheet material.

She said: 'Either I get physical pains in certain places, and I am worried about my health, or if the physical pains are not there, I have this general feeling of tension everywhere. I have read almost every book on earth that has any bearing, physical or mental, upon this subject, and all I realize from my reading is that the whole thing is imagination. But that does not prevent me from feeling tensions and panics. It is as though when a pain comes, my brain goes. I live in a world of people who, if they knew I had come to consult you, would think I was completely mad. I take sedatives at night to make me sleep.'

Still respecting her defences and resistances, I then took the opportunity at this interview to obtain some outline of family history and past history. When we came to her father, she ejaculated the remark, which I noted for further reference: 'He's the cause of all my trouble. He wanted a boy, and I was a girl. I came to know that I didn't satisfy him. Very early in life I had to face up to the fact that he was not fond of me. That was a real blow.'

This presently led to the story of the shock her father gave her when she was *six* years of age. She said: 'I was with my mother and father visiting some friends. An old gentleman there sat me on his knee, and said to my father, 'What a nice little girl you have here.' My father replied: 'I'm sorry I could not bring her sister. You should see her; she's a much finer child.' I cried all that night, and kept saying to myself, 'I'm *not* jealous of my sister.' At first the patient did not know which came first, the sexual phantasy-habit which she called 'masturbation', or this psychological shock from her father's remark.

She has throughout clung to the conviction that if her parents had really loved her, and shown her love, her tensions would have disappeared, and the 'masturbatory' habit would either never have developed, or would have disappeared. She said: 'It was the unhappiness all through my childhood, owing to my feeling that they didn't love me, which produced the tension, and it was the tension that produced the habit.'

Furthermore, she declared that her parents were always prodding her and trying to drive her to scholastic success—according to her as a means to their own aggrandizement. She said: 'Every time I attempted a real mental effort, it simply increased my tension, and led to the "masturbation" experience with involuntary orgasm. So how could I be expected to be first in the class? Nobody, not even my mother, ever suspected that anything like this was going on in me.'

Apparently the automatic process, including the orgasm, was a necessary physiological or pathological mechanism, acquired by her body and nervous system for the purpose of reducing the tension. There is evidence that all psychoneurotic symptoms may be so regarded. In short, it would seem that if we do not voluntarily discover and utilize means of discharging or reducing our accumulating nervous tension, some automatic process within the body, something perhaps phylogenetically older, unconscious and involuntary, will take over the job itself, whether we consciously desire it or not. Psychogenic visceral disturbances come under this category, perhaps no less than did this woman's particular symptom. Indeed, we may regard all our activities, social or otherwise, all our reaction formations, and even our beliefs and attitudes of mind, as, as it were, 'symptomatic' expressions of a natural process of discharge of dynamic energy or reduction of tension.

E*

CHAPTER XXI

THE HISTORY AND NATURE OF HER PRINCIPAL SYMPTOM

THERE is a difference, but not necessarily a fundamental difference, between processes to which we consent voluntarily, or even promote voluntarily, and those which take place involuntarily in spite of ourselves. Admittedly the latter are more apt to be called symptoms. Nevertheless, there is a good deal of justification for the term 'symptomatic behaviour', however voluntary such behaviour may be.

Even at the first interview with the patient I have just been discussing a certain amount of the aetiology of her principal symptom was revealed. However true or untrue her theory may be that, had she received adequate demonstrations of love from her parents, her tension would have been sufficiently low to obviate the development of her symptom, there is certainly some evidence that it began very early indeed. She remembered what she thinks may have been her first undoubted orgasm occurring at the age of about seven. She says her governess was telling her a story of a punishment the governess had received at her convent school when she was a little girl. For the very petty 'crime' of secretly nibbling off a corner of her lunch-time slab of chocolate, the governess had been made to stand immobile in the centre of the playground during the play interval, while the other girls played around her, some of them jeering at her. The governess related how, as a child, recognizing the alleged enormity of her guilt, she had *acquiesced* in this punishment. At that point my patient, aged seven, had experienced a complete involuntary orgasm.

Subsequently she remembered how, when she was at a kindergarten class from the age of four years, she had been completely preoccupied with the minor punishments which the infants around her were, it seems, frequently receiving. She said: 'When I was at the kindergarten school at five years of age, I was in a state of excitement all the time. When any child was put in a corner, I felt this same tense emotional feeling, and an impulse to masturbate. I was always excited by children being punished, and the excitement was always accompanied by a physical sensation, a sort of thrill all over my body, but I don't think it actually amounted to orgasm until the occasion of the governess's story when I was seven. Every day at the kindergarten school I was in a state of excitement at the prospect of one of these stupid little punishments taking place. Later on I learnt to check my enjoyment of it at the time, and to treasure the memory of it to enjoy that night when I was at home in bed. I think that is how I learned to make it purely a mental process.

'All through my childhood, the other thing that obsessed me was an anxiety to win the praise or approval of my mother and father. Punishment was the last thing that I wanted for myself. It was their love that I wanted all the time. I realize now that the silly people thought it was bad for me to show me any love. They put on this act of disparagement, thinking, I suppose, it would make me better, whereas actually it has ruined my whole life, and destroyed my health.'

There are several comments one can make in connection with this material if only to prevent it from being unduly misleading. One is that there may be something in this patient's contention that a demonstration of parental love would have saved her from all her trouble. I shall refer to this again at the end, though one should say at the moment, that there appears to be a strong bias on the part of people suffering from psychoneurosis to blame their parents for their illness. Hatred of parents is a symptom which commonly emerges in the course of analysis. But it would appear that some parents who behaved very badly had children who grew up relatively normal, whereas others, who made only the usual and familiar mistakes, ('Every unanalysed adult can be guaranteed to treat a neurotic or a child inappropriately'), never cease to be vituperatively assailed by their psychoneurotic offspring. I should not say 'never cease to be assailed,' because one of the signs of successful analysis is when the patient ceases to hate and to blame his parents. Analysis reveals that this quarrel with the parents is a regressive projection (or regression) of the conflict between id and super-ego, the intrapsychic conflict behind every psychoneurosis.

Another point I should mention is that probably the *form* this patient's symptom took is not the most crucial matter. The most crucial matter is the fact that she had this extraordinary degree of tension. In consequence of this her mind, subconsciously at least, must have been casting about for some means of relief. She did not at that time suffer from migraine, from diarrhoea and vomiting, or other psychogenic visceral disturbances. (It is interesting to note that she had all these things later—when she inhibited the frequency of masturbatory relief). She found a mechanism or formation for the relief of her tensions suggested to her by the phenomenon of the punishments she witnessed in the nursery class. In other words, she seized upon this form because it came under her notice as part of her experience, and was utilizable for her unconscious purpose, namely for the relief of tension. If she had never witnessed such things as the punishments of children, it is conceivable that she would have found other ways or means of obtaining relief, perhaps more physiological and less mental. Unfortunately it was a form that led to progressive resistance to her natural indulgence in it. It was probably this resistance, more than anything else, which, depriving her of the only method of reduction of tension which she could utilize, caused her, in consequence, to suffer an undue degree of unrelieved and bottled-up tension.

This unrelieved tension then found physiological expression in the tenseness of her abdomenal muscles and in certain other physical and mental symptoms. One of the latter was the mental feeling, or thought, that some disaster was imminent. She would only have to get some little pain, probably psychogenic, that is to say caused by a contraction of muscle or viscera due to unrelieved tension, and she would immediately rationalize her mental feeling and idea of impending disaster, by linking it on to the physical pain, and feeling convinced that it was the worst of all possible things, namely cancer. Thus, her tension was expressing itself in various ways, physically and mentally.

To return to her theory that parental love would have either prevented or cured everything, evidence of some truth in it lies in the following. This patient, doubtless by virtue of telling me such tensely bottled-up secrets about herself, and also by virtue of her emotionally pressing need for a good-parent-image, soon achieved an outsize transference to me. She told me afterwards that, at and immediately after her first interview with me, her symptoms miraculously disappeared, and she felt that health and happiness were at last within her grasp. Of course, this proved to be an over-estimation, but it does indicate a relationship between transference, interpretable as emotional relationship to the parent image, and symptom-formation. It indicates that if the former is satisfactory, or seems to promise satisfaction, the latter does not take place.

Finally, I should admit that we have been dealing more with mechanisms than with the most fundamental or most primary source of things. The question, at the first interview, remained unanswered as to why this particular individual should have been selected by a 'maligant fate' to have such a degree of uncomfortable tension that symptoms had to be manufactured during earliest infancy. Was it an inherited factor, or was it something that occurred after birth? A suggestive answer to this conundrum is the information, subsequently received, that not only was she not breast-fed, but that from birth she suffered from definite digestive disturbances. These evidently continued until she was two years old, for at that age she was taken to a great specialist in diseases of children. He organized very special methods of feeding for her, to which, it is said, she owes her survival.

Are we then dealing with a trouble the cause of which lies so far back in earliest infancy (from birth) that nothing can be expected to ameliorate it? Against this suggestion we have not only the fact that this patient's capacity for transference is so great, but also the fact that removal of negative elements of her transference by interpretation, without the complete dissolusion of positive elements, leads to sufficient amelioration to make all the difference between intolerable discomfort with ill health and a considerable degree of happiness, though not yet entirely symptom-free.

For those who are interested, I am tempted to describe the psychopathological composition of this patient's principal symptom, despite the likelihood that some readers will not be able to accept it.

To begin on general lines, one can say that an infant, like any other living organism, is born with certain inherited patterns called instincts. Some are already operative at birth; others will reveal themselves only at a later stage of maturation. Now instincts are inherited paths along which the organism discharges its tensions. The successful discharge of these tensions is accompanied by a feeling of relief, called gratification. All is well and the pleasure-principle operates satisfactorily so long as instincts can proceed towards their aim, namely towards gratification. It is only when there is frustration to this smooth process that tension reaches a pitch which is accompanied by increasing discomfort, eventually intolerable discomfort. To my mind this is identical with a state of anxiety or at least with some primitive equivalent of anxiety.

Amongst the first regular interferences with the infant's gratification of its instincts is the interference of the parents. The parents begin, sooner or later, to demand that the child shall please them, shall conform to their desires, rather than obey the sole autonomy of its instincts. The tension which this interference or frustration provokes can only be relieved by some alternative form of gratification. Normally this becomes that of satisfaction in pleasing the parents, and, thereby, winning their love, which brings with it a sense of security. This, in turn, has a great deal to do with mitigating the feelings of anxiety set up by the original instinct-frustration. We must note, however, that before this change has been achieved, a certain amount of conflict has been experienced and suffered by the organism. Thus, from this material, one can see how important it could have been for this patient to feel that she was loved by her parents. The only alternative to the gratification of being loved by her parents and the accompanying feelings of security, would be that of the original direct relief of instinct-tension. It seems pretty clear that in this case the patient became the victim of very considerable conflict. This caused her to turn at one moment to relief of tension by instinct gratification, and, at another moment, to strenuous attempts to curtail this in favour of gratifying her parents, and winning their love, a love which they appeared to be so reluctant to give her. It only remains to add that before we are justified in calling this state of affairs 'conflict' in the psychological sense, we are assuming that the parents, or rather their mental effects upon the child, have been introjected into the child's mind to form the super-ego. The intrapsychic conflict is between the child's id on the one hand and its super-ego (plus ego) on the other.

This is, to my mind, a classical or standard description of the earliest state of conflict at what is called a 'structural level' of mental development. How can it be resolved? It can be resolved only if a certain amount of instinct gratification can at the same time be coupled with the acquired desire or imperative need to reach security by pleasing the parents. Thus, the instinct levels of the child and the acquired need to gain love and security from its parents, must to some extent be brought into line with each other. That alone can resolve conflict and lead to satisfactory adjustment.

A *full* understanding of this patient's psycho-pathology can only be arrived at if we, first of all, consider the details of the phantasy through which she obtained relief. The standard or classical form of this phantasy was briefly as follows:

A girl of some importance, a girl whom she admired, had committed some fault or crime; an older woman, usually a teacher, whom she also admired and loved, was taxing the girl with this crime, and explaining to her that she would have to be punished for it. It was essential that the older woman loved the girl. Thus, she explained to the girl that it was for the girl's own good that this punishment had to be done. Invariably the climax, or near climax, of the phantasy came when the girl herself acknowledged her guilt, acquiesced in the punishment, and voluntarily surrendered to it. It was at this point, or upon further progress of this phantasy, that the patient obtained orgasm.

In the light of what I have said about the conflict between instinct-levels (or id) on the one hand, and parental edicts (super-ego) on the other hand, perhaps the reader can see that the delinquent girl in the phantasy represented symbolically the *id* part of the conflict, and that the punisher or teacher represented the *super-ego*. In the culprit's admission of guilt and acquiescence in the punishment we have, as it were, some sort of union or reconciliation between id and super-ego.

Nevertheless, there are several things which still remain unsolved. One is the nature of the crime or delinquency which the girl has committed. Another is the symbolical significance of the punishment which the teacher demanded that the girl should accept, and in which the girl finally acquiesced.

Now, both these questions were answered or solved in the course of the analysis of this patient's deeper unconscious mind. The answers will seem to the unanalysed reader very curious indeed and quite incredible. They were the parts of the phantasy which were repressed by the patient's mind, and are probably repressed by every normal unanalysed adult. That is why they are as mysterious and incredible as the symptom. Nevertheless, they are in strict conformity with the Freudian theory of the Oedipus complex. I cannot adduce anything like the evidence which this patient's clinical material presented. I can produce only the conclusions to which all the material, including her symptoms and dreams, pointed.

The symbolical significance of the punishment, coupled with the culprit's acquiescence, should I think be patent from the fact that it produced psychosexual orgasm. The nature of the crime may not be so obvious, until we reflect that the subconscious mind always 'makes the punishment fit the crime'. In this case it fitted so well that it was practically identical. The punishment was administered by a parent-figure, *and* it produced orgasm!

In short, the crime of the culprit was the Oedipus crime. She had displaced (destroyed) her mother (in her transference she constantly asked me if I was all right!) in the course of obtaining, or attempting to obtain, gratification from the father-image. It appears to make no difference that she was frustrated in her pursuit of the conscious-level equivalent of this aim, namely to get her father to take some notice of her, and to care for her. Apparently the crime was there nevertheless, and—worse than the crime—the continued frustration or deprivation of the needed gratification, the aim of her developing instinct. At the same time, it was essential, for security's sake, that she should have a reconciliation with the mother-image, as well as gratification from the father-image. Apparently, reconciliation with the mother-image could only be achieved through absolute and complete atonement for her crime. She had to acquiesce in the punishment.

If, as sometimes happened, orgasm did not arrive immediately on acquiescence, the phantasy had to continue, and a curious feature of its extended development was that the actual execution of the punishment was delegated by the woman schoolteacher to some man who had to perform it. If orgasm had not already arrived the punishment would proceed in the form of a beating on the hind quarters or buttocks, administered by this man delegated by the woman. There was clinical evidence to show that this act was a symbolical expression of her phantasy of a sexual relationship to her father. For instance, the whip used was none other than the dog-whip her father carried.

Thus, this patient's orgasm-giving phantasy represented symbolically the gratification of everything which her entire psyche needed. Within it were included, one, a gratification of her sexual instinct (id) by a symbolical anticipation or experience of the sexual act with the father-image, two, a reconciliation of the mother-image by atonement, and, three, a perfect solution of the conflict between id and super-ego by combining the satisfaction of both sides of her psyche—inherited instinct pattern (id) and introjected parent (super-ego)—in the same symbolical act of punishment.

In short, every level or facet of her psyche was satisfied by this phantasy, conflict was resolved, and complete gratification, with orgasm, attained. Small wonder that in these circumstances the phantasy had persisted throughout her life as a method of relieving the accumulating tensions which nothing else appeared to relieve. Without this resolution one side of her frustrated the other side, and no side obtained satisfaction. All she had was a perpetual conflict with its accompanying unrelieved tension. By the wonderful device of getting her 'id' to acquiesce in her super-ego-ordered punishment, she not only atoned for her crime, but was, at the same time, seducing her super-ego (parent) into performing for her the very act (sexual intercourse) for the crime of which she was atoning. Thus, all 'parties' were reconciled, and all 'parties' were simultaneously gratified by the same act. It was, therefore, from an intrapsychic point of view, an ideal solution; it resolved all the conflicts and relieved all the accumulated tensions, purely by virtue of the intrapsychic processes which took place during the phantasy. No wonder that, once discovered, her psyche continued to use this device throughout her life.

The only disadvantage of it was that with the development of her ego and its increasing need for reality-contact and adjustment, this retreat into introverted phantasy failed to satisfy her increasing reality-factor. She, her ego at least, wanted a real personal human relationship for its gratification, and this, to be satisfactory and complete, would have to be capable of embodying the whole of her emotional potentialities, including the sexual. Her transference has shown that it was lack of reciprocal rapport with her parents which denied her this full normal personal adjustment, and substituted for it a fixation to childhood phantasy, with consequent frigidity in intercourse. Her transference has shown too that this is all remediable. Analysis reveals to her that the old phantasies are, not only absent, but impossible to invoke during sessions solely *because* she has a *much greater interest* in the personal relationship between her analyst and herself. This interest supercedes everything else . . . there are no punishment phantasies, no symptoms, no tensions.

The position is one of anticipation of an harmonious union of super-ego (parent, analyst) and id (her emotional need), perhaps a return to that pre-conflict stage of life when unadulterated and all-gratifying love prevailed between parent (subsequent super-ego) and 'innocent' infant (id), the stage before the Pandora box was opened and her happy id-life overshadowed by the evil clouds of hateful frustration, prohibition, guilt, pain and punishment. She can feel that, through analysis, harmony will come again into her intrapsychic world and give her the opportunity of playing it out successfully in her reality contacts. When super-ego and id are reconciled, and the psyche no longer a house divided against itself, the ego should have little difficulty in gaining the co-operation of reality, of environment and its personal contacts, to project, dramatize, make real and external, the happy (i.e. gratifying) condition that is already being experienced internally.

PARTS III TO V: PRACTICE

PART FOUR

'GUYS AND DOLLS'

CHAPTER XXII

SEXUALLY INHIBITED MEN

IN the course of one's professional work as a psychiatrist and psychotherapist, one interviews a seemingly infinite variety of human beings of both sexes, and conducts a course of analysis or psychotherapy in a large number of cases. There are as many varieties of people who come for consultation or treatment as there are of people who never come.

Our attention in this book is focused upon the proclivity for personal contacts and relationships of a variety of people, and the degree of emotional interest or response which accompanies these relationships. In my opinion it is impossible or artificial to make a general classification of people with any degree of rigidity, whether they be sufferers from psychological trouble, or so-called normal persons; but in respect of personal relationships, there does appear to be a gradation from the incredibly inhibited to what might seem to be the incredibly uninhibited. I should add this qualification: with regard even to the apparently uninhibited, so far as people who consult a therapist are concerned, they practically always turn out to be people with an inhibition at some less visible, some more fundamental level, for instance an inhibition which results in some degree of orgastic deficiency. In other words, they are people whose relationship to others is free enough to include even what appears to be a normal sexual life, until one discovers that orgastic relief in their sexual relationship is absent or inadequate. Thus, even such cases fit the old-standing theory that neurosis or neurotic symptoms are manufactured out of a libidinal residue that fails to achieve psychosexual discharge.

Be that as it may, the theory of the psychogenic precipitation of nervous illness is still well established. It is briefly as follows: First, there is a frustration, or inhibition, of adequate libidinal satisfaction. (*Normally* satisfaction is characteristic of a complete heterosexual personal relationship.) Second, libido being frustrated in this natural movement towards the achievement of its aim (psychosexual orgasm), *regresses*, and, in the course of its regression, re-activates *component instincts*, particularly at points where there was some temporary libidinal arrest or *fixation*. In other words, if an individual has, in the course of development, been unduly long fixated at some earlier stage of sexual development, such as phallic (including clitorid) urethral, anal, or oral, his libido, if frustrated from a mature genital-personal gratification, will tend to regress to his particular fixation point, and to re-activate the pleasures, conscious or unconscious, which he formerly enjoyed most at an earlier stage of his development.

The next aetiological factor in the production of neurosis is that the enjoyment of such a component instinct, e.g. in the form of a perversion, meets with resistance from the super-ego and ego. Conflict arises. If the opposition to libidinal discharge at this component instinct level is sufficient to cause *repression* of the desires, and of the conflict, from consciousness, there may result a situation sufficiently full of dynamic energy to force a discharge in some displaced direction. This direction may be mental or visceral. The resulting symptom includes elements from both sides of the conflict, derivatives of libido, and derivatives of the opposing and repressing forces.

In the meantime, through the process of regression, earlier and earlier stages of emotional development and their attendant conflicts or complexes, are re-activated. This process primarily goes back to what is known as the Oedipus complex. As a result, the individual is largely preoccupied, whether he knows it or not, with the emotional pattern of early infancy, pertaining to a stage where frustration was insurmountable, and where phantastic desires encountered equally phantastic fears of punishment. The aggressive or death instinct is, in my opinion, largely reactive to frustration, especially at this stage of development. It is, of course, very much subject to projection. In other words, it is sensed as not belonging to the self, but as an attribute of the punishing parent or super-ego, and this leads to the extraordinarily excessive fear of retribution.

All these things are going on under the surface, probably in every person we meet, but more especially or more conspicuously in those suffering from nervous trouble. It is the struggle under the surface which affects and determines the emotional reactions to personal relationship in the individual. There can be an almost infinite variety of such reactions. In the light of this material, so-called normal persons can be seen to be, for the most part, just another variety or degree of morbidly inhibited people.

Passing in review a series of men patients, from the most obviously inhibited to the apparently uninhibited, I think first of a man in the late twenties, who was brought to see me by a very motherly looking mother. The story was almost incredible. He seemed quite surprised when I asked him if he had ever in his life had any girl friends. He said he had not had time. He was working for his father in a very active business. Of all the people I have met, other than psychotics, I think of this man as amongst the most sexually inhibited or retarded. He had never masturbated. He had never kissed a girl, except at Christmas parties. He had never had any emotional response to the opposite sex. One is usually right in assuming that such cases are repressed homo-sexuals, but in this instance there was absolutely no justification for such a theory.

One of the most curious features of the case was the fact that the inhibition of his sexuality had extended to physiological levels. Nocturnal emissions were not unknown, but he could hardly remember when the last one had occurred, 'probably something like three or six months ago'. Anyhow, this was enough to show that his endocrine glands at least, if not his mind, were capable of some sexual function.

The reason he was brought to me was on account of a number of phobias. One was his inability to travel unaccompanied. This explained why mother had accompanied him, but to my mind it was not the only explanation of her presence. In the light of his dreams, and other analytical material, it soon became clear that emotionally and psychosexually, he was still largely fixated to infancy, still living unconsciously in the emotional pattern and phantasy of his Oedipus complex. It was more than a mother-fixation. It was a love-life, so far as heterosexuality was concerned, confined to mother, with its inevitable total repression of genital sexuality.

The curious feature of this case was that, as repressive resis-tances weakened, as anxiety became sufficiently assuaged to lessen the absolute power of repression, his conduct in respect of his personal contacts developed in the direction of normality. Presently he even went so far as to accompany a party to a palais-de-danse, and before long he was, perhaps imitatively, actually dancing with girls whom he had never previously met. The first effect of this was that immediately he put his arm round a girl to dance, he experienced an automatic and violent erection (without phantasy). Before he had taken many steps on the dance floor he experienced ejaculation, the whole physiological process being so dissociated from his mind that, curiously enough, it did not worry him. It was as though something a little inconvenient happened which had nothing to do with him anyway!

However, these very morbid phenomena presently gave place to more normal modifications. It was only a question of time, barely a few months, before his functions on the dance floor were normal, and shortly after this he formed acquaintanceships with a succession of young women, and it was interesting to learn how each acquaintanceship made progress towards a greater and more normal emotional meaning. Long before it happened one was gratified to see that a normal heterosexual relationship would most certainly come about, normal on an emotional and on a physiological level. Simultaneously, all the psychoneurotic symptoms, including the phobias, disappeared. He had grown up from infancy to adolescence or maturity in an unusually short space of time.

Another man of about the same age told me at his first interview that the symptom for which he had come for treatment was nothing more or less than a slight stammer. I opened my eyes a little, and he added: 'You may not have noticed it.' I had not. He then tried to build up a case in favour of his theory that what he was suffering from was a stammer, but the most he could say for it was that when he was asked on the telephone suddenly to give his phone number, he would start with, 'Er.'

I asked him if he had any other symptoms, and at first he said 'No.' There were various theories as to why and how the stammer had come about. Then, as though inadvertently, he happened to mention that until recently he had been engaged to a girl. Two weeks ago they had broken it off, by mutual consent, but they were still seeing each other. He was rather a heterosexual looking type of person, and, as our interview did not seem to be getting on to anything very illuminating, I finally asked him whether he had ever had sexual intercourse. His reply was a little unusual. He said: 'No, not since I was thirteen years of age.'

By this time I had begun to suspect that, unknown to himself, this young man was probably psychosexually impotent, or very nearly so. And that was probably the explanation for his shilly-shallying over the engagement to his girl-friend. His remark that he had not had sexual intercourse since thirteen years of age naturally led to the story of his childhood sexuality. The characteristic of this was, or became, very clear. His emotional life was essentially at an Oedipus level, confined to his relationship to mother and father. Mother was the unfailing sexual stimulus, and the super-ego aspect of the parents, especially of father, but not excluding mother, was the stimulus for an enormous castration anxiety.

Here, I am naturally speaking of a state of affairs of which he was unconscious. He knew only of the manifestations thereof, and even that knowledge, when first it came, was far from being clear to him. The stammer he referred to was, of course, a derivative. It was nothing more than a symbol in consciousness, conjured up to represent the equivalent terrific 'stammer' in his unconscious of his psychosexual function. Consciously he told me that he stammered (which he did not). Unconsciously he was telling himself and me that he suffered from an anxiety which caused his sexual function, in so far as its object-relationship was concerned, to 'stammer'.

His unconscious emotional life was almost confined to his Oedipus complex. It was not so very long before it transpired that in his case he had, as an infant, been quite *conscious* of genital erotic feelings and desires actually towards his mother. He had also been quite conscious of their prohibition by fear, particularly by fear of his father. Very soon he remembered that he had tried to get out of this situation, which even at that age he had found pretty intolerable, by a displacement of the love object, or rather of the sexual aspect of the love object, from his mother on to a sister eighteen months younger than himself. He declares that he was only six and a half when he started making actual attempts at intercourse with his sister.

First of all, the story was of actual intercourse with his sister for a considerable number of years; but subsequently, as things grew clearer, it appeared that the conflict, or the anxiety of the conflict, which was still inhibiting his heterosexual potency, had not only apparently repressed his sexual phantasies regarding his mother, but had inhibited his attempted intercourse with this sister, and prevented his achieving potency with her. What he had experienced in this sexual relationship had very conspicuously been all stages of anxiety from the mildest to the most acute.

It was this pattern which still dominated his sexual life, and finally led to the same 'stammer' in his adult sexual function as had characterized his childhood sexual attempts. Nevertheless, this man's personal relationships were not so odd as might have been expected from a recital of this pattern. As with his mother, and with his younger sister, so with people in general, he had a libidinal or pleasure-driven urge to approach them, and to enjoy a friendly relationship with them. In exact correspondence with his childhood pattern, the inhibiting forces only became really anxiety-provoking and inhibiting if and when a relationship approached sexual intercourse.

CHAPTER XXIII

IMMATURE MEN

ANOTHER case of rather a different nature, but in this instance conspicuously characterized by defect in personal relationship, was that of a young man, again in the late twenties, who was unusually intelligent and well-educated.

At the first interview, he said to me: 'I am worried on account of a very deep-seated way of behaviour. It is a sort of negative way of behaving. I can give you two instances of what I mean. Recently I was engaged to be married. At a time when I was not in a position to marry the girl, I felt I wanted to marry her, but as soon as I was actually in a position to marry her, I found I didn't want to. It is not the first time something like that has happened to me.

'The other instance is in connection with work. I don't quite know what I want to be, so I am in a sort of meandering state. For a long time I thought I would *like* to be a writer, but although I was so keen on the idea of being a writer, I did not do anything about it. Well, I'm not quite speaking the truth when I tell you that. What I did do about it eventually was to take a bed-sitting room, and sit in it . . . and think about myself as a writer. I tried to write once or twice, but really didn't know what to write about!'

This proved to be a very complex and difficult case. One might say there was insufficient emotional drive in his life to get him anywhere, either with love (c.f. the engagement story), or with sex, or with people, or even for that matter with himself. 'Wanting to be a writer', not that he had anything to write, merely meant that he wanted the satisfaction of some contribution to his self-esteem or pride. On deeper analysis it appeared that, in spite of his intelligence, his emotional pattern was a very childish or infantile one. But saying that is not saying enough, for some children do have a considerable capacity for 'object love', or at least an emotional need for other people. This 'child' was more like the wolf who walks alone. His love object, his personal relationship, was essentially himself. Emotionally he did not really want or need any other person. Like the 'being a writer', it was just a phantasy to bolster up his self-esteem. So, it was very nice to be engaged, so long as one were not in a position actually to marry. To be actually married to a real woman would be a tragedy. What on earth would he want her for? The bit of sexuality, even if he were capable of it, would not be adequate to justify being tied to a person, an 'alien'. The only person he was really tied to was himself.

His unhappiness was superficially due to it being difficult to find enough in himself to be very happy about. At one stage he developed a phantasy that if he could gain success at anything, he would be happier. If there were any truth in this, it was only because he would then find some justification in admiring and loving himself, and he felt there would be satisfaction in that.

Of course, we do get more extreme cases of this form of so-called narcissistic neurosis. So far as personal relationships are concerned, they are characterized by the deficiency of such relationships, or the absence of a capacity for such relationships. Schizophrenia might be regarded as the last degree of this situation. There the individual withdraws from all object relationships, people and things, the whole world of reality, and lives entirely, or almost entirely, within his own phantasy life. On account of frustration this phantasy life has commonly regressed in the meantime to a very early infantile, pre-Oedipus level. The emotional development activating it is earlier than what is called the genital level of libidinal development.

It is from a multitude of observations such as these that the psycho-analytical theory has developed, that the earliest libidinal pleasures, from the oral level onwards, are essentially autoerotic. That is to say, at those primitive levels the infant is obtaining gratification from his physiological processes, without the need for any whole-object, such as a person in a personal relationship. The theory is that, it is only when libidinal development progresses to what is called a full genital level that 'whole-object' (or personal) relationship becomes a necessary ingredient of it.

This may be a difficult theory to understand unless one is professionally engaged in studying the subject, and analysing people suffering from various degrees of deficient emotional development, or people who, through frustration, have regressed to early fixation points.

For our purposes, in this book, the theory is of interest as suggesting that the unconscious emotional or sexual basis of an adequate personal relationship must be *a priore*, that the individual has, at some stage of his life, attained a full genital level of libidinal development. It is not that, prior to such a level (commonly supposed to be reached between the ages of three and five), the individual is unappreciative of his environment or of things in his environment, but that, from an emotional-interest point of view, they generally tend to be part-objects rather than whole-objects. What is meant by this is that prior to a genital level of development a 'thing' can be used for pleasure, but a person, a whole person, a personality, is not required as such. The erotic life is essentially autoerotic, rather than alloerotic or primarily concerned with the love of a person. Instruments or objects can be used for autoerotic purposes, for example, at an oral level, such an instrument as the mother's nipple, the teat of the bottle, one's own thumb, and, subsequently, all things which give oral pleasure, right up to and including things connected with eating, drinking, and smoking; but these do not involve personal relationships. They are part-object aids to autoerotic gratification.

Similarly I think, on reflection, it may be evident to us that a lot of relationships, masquerading as personal relationships in some people's love life, are, if the truth were known, more part-object relationships similarly contributing to autoerotic pleasure. For instance, a man who uses a 'nice body' for his erotic enjoyment is, psychologically speaking, to my mind, using a part-object for autoerotic genital gratification.

This brings us to the subject of fetishism and perversions in general. They are instances of the use of part-objects for sexual pleasure. And, in so far as they are this, they are using up libido, in a sense, autoerotically, and detracting from the quantity of libido left available for whole-object personal relationships. On this account people excessively subject to them, even without our having a knowledge of their proclivities, are commonly less satisfactory in personal relationships than is the emotionally mature person.

Without being psychologists we all learn to sense their unsatisfactoriness. I should add though that even here there can be all sorts of proportions, variations, and admixtures. I would like to add further that so-called normal persons are by no means entirely free from this blemish in their capacity for whole-object love and full personal relationships. Otherwise, why should a girl have to frizz herself up to win her man, and why should the town be full of shops selling dresses and personal ornament? It is normal to be to some degree 'abnormal' in this respect and to get a good deal of our 'love'-excitement from the 'perversion' of fetishistic stimulation.

The fact may seem curious to those who are not psychologists or psycho-analysts that people who do not require another person for their pleasure, for the purpose of their libidinal satisfaction, in general do not have an adequate rapport to other persons. It is as though the individual, the person as such, is not necessary to them. The person they are with, whom they are forced into some sort of contact with, usually feels this sooner or later.

This is relevant to the answer I give when a patient says to me: 'I always masturbate a great deal, Doctor; is there any harm in it? It used to be said that it was a very bad thing for one's nerves, that it produced nervous illness, and worse, but I have heard that the modern idea is that it does no harm whatsoever. Is that true?'

My reply to such a question is this: 'Those who get their sexual satisfaction by masturbating are obviously independent of a sexual partner, and so rather independent of society, of relationships to other people—as well as, of course, of a particular relationship to a particular person for sexual reasons, or for any other reasons.' So I say to such patients: 'If you persist in masturbation, you will find that you require less and less the intimate company of any other person; therefore, masturbation will tend to make you something of a recluse.'

Now, that is in keeping with what I have just said, that those who do not require another person for their libidinal satisfaction tend to lose not only a sexual partner—they tend to go through life without a sexual partner—but they also tend to go through life with less and less personal contact. Such personal contacts as they do have are, in a sense, somewhat impersonal.

In the same way, those who are fetishistically inclined, such, for instance, as hair fetishists, are very much attracted to their fetish, to a beautiful head of hair, or to the particular type of hair which happens to be their special attraction; in consequence, they are not, to the same extent as a normal person, attracted to the person as a whole. They may even marry a beautiful head of hair, but they may neglect the character, temperament, various requirements and so on of the other individual. In short, they may not be reacting to the emotional life, the emotional reactions, of the other individual. Thus, their wives, and everyone else in intimate relationship with them, find them unsatisfactory persons, emotionally empty, as far as the other party is concerned. When you come to think of it, why should they be otherwise? They are not interested in the other party, or in the other party's emotional reactions, at least not to the same extent as is the normal, mature person. Their interest is taken up with the hair instead, with something which is called in psycho-analysis, a part-object. Similarly, fetishists or perverts who like some particular practice, such as flagellation, would be interested in the other person from that point of view. In so far as the other person is not a similar pervert, their interest is defective in that respect, and, indeed, in every respect that matters to the other person.

Generally speaking, perverts, fetishists, and other sexually abnormal people are re-living their component-instinct level of sexuality. As I have said, anything short of, anything more immature than, the full genital level of sexuality is characterized by attachment to a part-object rather than to a whole-object, or to a personality. Perverts, and, to some extent, most neurotics, will have contact along certain lines with similar proclivities in their partners, but, something will be lacking as regards a full personal relationship; and, if the other person is sexually mature, and therefore requires a full personal relationship, the other person will find such people unsatisfactory, or not wholly satisfactory, perhaps more like one would find children. One cannot be satisfied all one's life with such a mate.

These characteristics of people who are not fully mature naturally reveal themselves during the course of an analysis, but my point in this book is to suggest that very often such things can be sensed, even at an interview. Perhaps they can be sensed, by some people at any rate, during the first few moments of conversation after an introduction. Sooner or later, if not during the first few moments, the mature person will begin to wonder about the other, or perhaps just vaguely feel that the other person is not wholly satisfactory as a companion or friend. In other words, the immature person, whether neurotic, perverted, fetishistic, or simply without a full capacity for personal relationship, such as one gets in inveterate masturbators, is felt to be emotionally lacking in some sense or another, however 'over-sexed', in a sense, he or she may be as regards his or her particular perversion or sexual addiction.

Something similar is the case with homosexuals. But there, of course, we often have an excessive personal or intimate relationship with the personality of the particular member of the same sex to whom the homosexual is attracted. Like the fetishist with his 'hair' for instance, the homosexual has his whole emotional life absorbed in his homosexual attraction. The person towards whom he is homosexually attracted, if also a homosexual, and similarly attracted towards him, will find him just everything. But, when he spends any appreciable time in the company of a normal woman, she will find him just nothing. The point I am trying to make is that she will not find him just nothing, merely in a sexual sphere, she will find him emotionally uninteresting, and generally uninteresting, somehow unsatisfactory. She will feel more or less as though she were alone when he is in her company. Of course, he will feel similarly uninterested. It is the sexual attraction, the particular variety and nature of it, which lies at the basis of personality attraction, of the interest of one person in another (however unconscious the sexual element may be) and of one person's capacity to arouse reciprocal interest in another person. These interests need not be consciously sexual, but they are, none the less, the basis of a personal relationship.

CHAPTER XXIV

PERVERTED MEN

A NUMBER of excerpts from my clinical work, interviews, psycho-therapeutic treatments, and analyses, occur to me. They will help to illustrate and give point to these remarks.

For instance, I once had a patient who told me he was a hair fetishist. Although married, and with a family of young children, he would, nevertheless, on his way home from work, occasionally be seized with a compulsion to follow his fetishistic interest. He would wait about in crowds, looking for a woman with the particular type of hair which he found so attractive and stimulating. Having found her, he would endeavour to get his face as close to her hair as possible, with due regard, of course, to not getting himself into trouble as a public nuisance. Unbeknown to the woman he would then indulge in the most exciting sexual feelings and phantasies. These manoeuvres commonly led to his following her, or sitting next to her in public vehicles, and so on, sometimes for hours on end.

In the meantime, his poor wife and family were sitting at home, expecting him, and wondering why he was getting so late. Obviously his interest in the fetishistic object, in this head of hair, detracted from his interest and happiness with his wife and family. They lost what his fetishistic attraction gained. Libidinally, of course, his phantasy was to get closer and closer to this head of hair. What he would have liked, and what he occasionally achieved, was to get a sufficiently good relationship to the woman carrying the head of hair, to enable him to stroke it, to comb it, to brush it. This was to him far more sexually exciting than intercourse with his wife, or than any ordinary sexual intercourse.

On the other hand, his perversion naturally caused him a great deal of conflict. That is why he came for treatment. He wanted, and his super-ego wanted him, to be a good, faithful, loving husband; but here was this thing pulling him away. He confessed to me that there was more duty than pleasure in being a good husband. Following the fetish, on the other hand, was pure pleasure, and, of course, the antithesis of duty. Hence the conflict. In some respects, perhaps in fundamental, emotional, instinctual respects, he could have done without his wife and family, and they, poor things, of course felt it. His wife felt that she was married to only part of a man. And the part she did have was characteristically secretive and defensive. I myself felt it at the first interview. He was reserved, careful, still and stilted—even in his physical movements. Not the least of his troubles arose from his excessively guilt-ridden attitude to his addiction. Men with a comparable addiction to golf or to gambling do not feel so guilty.

In connection with the psychology of the homosexual, and the deficiency of his heterosexual personal relationship, the following surprising little incident occurs to me: A patient had presented himself because, he said, he wanted very keenly indeed—and he was ready to implement his statement by paying for treatment— to be cured of his homosexual proclivities, and to become, instead, heterosexual. He rightly said, homosexuality held no future as regards companionship in one's later life. Also, he claimed that he had detected in himself a certain, though slight, proclivity for heterosexual relationships. As you will see from the story, he was perhaps over-optimistic, or boasting a little, when he made this claim. Another peculiarity about him, perhaps in this case not so peculiar, was the fact that his sexuality was much aroused by listening to good music.

After he had been coming to me for some weeks, he was relating the experiences he had had the evening before the session. He said: 'I was at a concert, and I enjoyed the music so much that I felt at the end of the performance that I must go out and find a companion; so I went to one of the large railway stations, and picked up a man. We went for a walk together, but, after I had been with him about half an hour, I realized that I did not care about him. So I got rid of him, dropped him, and went back to the station, and picked up another man. This one I liked quite well, and we got on, and finally went home together.'

The patient paused, expecting me to make some comment, so I said to him: 'You are coming to me with the alleged purpose of being made more heterosexual and less homosexual. Seeing that you were so romantically and sexually stirred up by the music and felt you must have some romantic or sexual affair, when you left the concert why on earth didn't you go out and pick up a woman, if you must pick up somebody, instead of a man?' This question of mine so astounded the patient that he sat up, turned round, and stared at me in bewilderment. 'What!' he said—as though the thought had never occurred to him before, as though I had suggested that he should perform some miracle, jump over the moon or something—'What!' he said, 'Me? Go out and pick up a *woman!*' He was silent for a time. Then he said: 'Good Heavens, Doctor, I wouldn't have a clue.'

In short, this man's sexual, emotional, and personal interests were such that he had no difficulty in doing what the average man would find extremely difficult, if not impossible, to accomplish—that is to say, to go into a strange place, look about, and find a strange man, get into conversation with him, and get into a sexual relationship with him. I venture to think, however, that the average heterosexual man, if emotionally pressed, as this person was after the concert, would find comparatively little difficulty in picking up somebody of the opposite sex. This patient had as little clue as to how to pick up a woman as the heterosexual man would have as to how to pick up a man. You can depend upon it that his personal relationship with people of the opposite sex was similarly deficient.

One might add that in the case of some homosexuals at least, their personal relationship to persons of the same sex as themselves is relatively greater, more dynamic, more emotional, more real, than that of the heterosexual person to either sex. I am suggesting here that the personal relationship follows the pattern of the sexual relationship, and can be a sublimation of it, particularly if there are difficulties in the way of its direct indulgence—as there often are in adult homosexuality—provided its potential energy is not unduly repressed.

In these chapters I started with a reference to the sexually inhibited and the sexually subnormal or defective patient. My intention was to proceed, through gradations of increasing sexual potentiality, to patients whose principal symptom appeared to be what might be called 'excessive sexuality'. Perverts and inveterate masturbators often appear to be over-sexed. For that matter, so do boys at puberty, and a number of adolescents. But I think, in many cases, the truth is different from the appearances.

An outstanding example of such a misleading impression is the case of the so-called nymphomaniac woman. Her characteristic symptom, the characteristic symptom of nymphomania, is that she must have one man after another—men, men, and men, all the time. It is as though she cannot have enough sex. Nothing will satisfy her. Well, the truth is just that—nothing *will* satisfy her. And the reason for it is not excessive sexuality, but some inhibition or defect in her sexuality. One characteristic, perhaps *the* characteristic, of the nymphomaniac woman is that she cannot achieve orgasm. That is why she has to keep on having sex, and sex again. It is just that, that she cannot reach satisfaction. Hence, her appetite is unsatisfied, perpetually unsatisfied, and she has produced a symptom, the characteristic feature of which is incessant attempts to satisfy that which cannot be satisfied. The reason it cannot be satisfied is not that she is over-sexed, but that she is orgastically inhibited. Thus, we might say that, in spite of the appearances of her behaviour, she is, scientifically speaking, not over-sexed but under-sexed.

Something similar is true of perverts and other people who appear to be indulging, or trying to indulge in an undue amount of sexuality—so called sex-obsessed people. A lot of them are going about in a sort of tumescent state, a state in which they are full of excitement, possibly almost at an acme of excitement, but never quite at the acme; they can never achieve the acme; they can never gain the full satisfaction which would bring them to rest. Everything stimulates, but the stimulation never reaches the point which can be called critical, and bring its reduction of tension. This can be a psychological difficulty as much as a physiological one.

The psychology of the Don Juan, for instance, can be as follows. Although he may, like most males, have no difficulty in achieving orgasm—orgasm and ejaculation—it does not bring him the full psychosexual satisfaction which a man capable of normal love would achieve in intimacy with his loved one. Generally speaking, he is a man with an unconscious mother-fixation, and, in his unconscious phantasy, he is wanting, and is spending his whole life, perhaps, in trying to achieve, the satisfaction (unconscious in form) which was denied him in infancy. He is unconsciously looking for the mother because his phantasy tells him that it is only with this special person that he will achieve the full satisfaction, the full joy, for which he has craved throughout his life. Perhaps practically every woman with whom he has not been intimate, every woman who is, as it were, at a distance, sexually, from him, is, thereby, made, by his unconscious phantasy, into a possible, a potential, mother. His instinct, as it were, feels that she is *the one;* but, no sooner does he achieve intimacy with her, than the experience, perhaps the very fact that he has had sexual access to her, makes her no longer the one. The thing has failed, like all his previous attempts. But, as the whole set-up is an unconscious one, that does not prevent him, not in the slightest, from feeling that the next woman, the next stranger, is the one, or *possibly* the one. He must have that one, and so it goes on and on.

I remember a patient who had an enormous reputation, or notoriety, in his particular circle, of being a terribly over-sexed man. This patient told me the following story. It was part of his reason for coming for analysis, so he said. His proclivities led him into a fairly gay social life, in some people often an effective substitute for sexuality. The story he told me was that he had, the previous evening, been to one of his frequent cocktail parties. There, across the crowded room, he had seen a beautiful young woman. She was the one, just the one that he wanted. He hardly thought these thoughts consciously; it so came about that he *felt* them. The next moment he saw that the woman talking to this young lady was somebody whom he knew. He realized that he only had to edge his way through the crowd, to these two, and the lady who knew him would introduce him to the beautiful girl whom he had just seen for the first time.

Now, while he was approaching the pair, an extraordinary thought occurred to him. It suddenly came to him with the vividness of a revelation. It was that only a few months ago he had been in an exactly similar situation. He had the familiar *déjà vu* experience. The essential difference was that the girl he knew, whom he anticipated would perform the introduction, had been, on that previous occasion, the unknown lovely. He had edged his way towards her, and been introduced. Some months had passed since then, and in the meantime everything had happened between them, including the cooling off and the parting.

But, the point was that, with this realization, came a far wider and more far-reaching one; and that was that throughout his life, since puberty, or at least since adolescence, similar things had been going on. He had been activated sexually all the time by this pursuit. Again and again it had happened, exactly as it was in process of happening at that very moment. What could he do about it? Was it a good thing? Was it a bad thing? Anyhow, it was a compulsion, he said, something apparently stronger than his own common sense or reason, which dragged him from one anticipation of delight to another, and from one danger to another—and from one worry to another. Was he going to go on like this all his life? Had he better come and do something about it? After all, he was now of a much more mature age than when it started. He was nearly forty, and it was still going on. Whatever would happen in his old age? Would he be left high and dry, without this urge, without companionship and without love?

However, the purpose of my story was to stress that these over-sexed individuals are not necessarily over-sexed in the sense of being more sexually mature than the average person. Their characteristic is usually, on the contrary, that they are somewhat immature sexually. You might say, if you like, that their sexuality has the vigour of youth. Well, there may be something in that, but it has also the inhibitions and the unsatisfactoriness of the emotions of youth. It has the compulsive quality, something outside the ego, of the emotional life of youth that does not bring the peace that mature, integrated sexuality brings. Very often in such persons, Don Juans or wolves, one finds the curious mixture of immature sexual tendencies combined with what appears to be the whole-object seeking. All sorts of perversions are sometimes mixed up in it too, though not very necessarily or very obviously.

In general, I think there is usually an excess of fetishistic attraction. Perhaps the whole-person, the new person, the girl they have never seen before, is more a fetish for their sexuality than a person. Often they do not really want to know *her*. They do not want to know her nature, except in so far as is necessary to achieve their sexual objective with a minimum of danger to themselves. They do not share with her psychologically. They just want something relatively superficial and immature. and then they are sick of it. Their sexuality has not achieved a mature adjustment with the social scheme of things, with the happiness of marriage and family. And that is to do with the fact that it is not altogether a whole-person object-relationship. Thus, in a sense, however over-sexed they may appear to be, it would be truer to say that they are under-sexed, at least in the sense of not being fully mature and integrated sexually.

There is commonly also, though not always, a certain amount of obvious boyish attitude and behaviour. To their sexual partner they will never be so satisfactory as the normal person, or they will not continue to be so. How could they be when they or their sexuality is not entirely satisfactory to themselves? Something is missing, perhaps the essential thing. A lot of stimulation, excite-ment and so on, goes on in their lives, but what is it all about? Excitement is, generally speaking, an anticipation of a satisfaction, something that will bring us to rest, contented, satisfied. That is what they never achieve, and that is why, like the nymphomaniac, they go from pillar to post, without actually getting anywhere.

However, do not let us make the mistake of blaming people for their sexual and personality development, or absence of it. The truth is that they are products of nature, their heredity and their circumstances, and are merely as it were the mouthpiece of what has been put into them.

Naturally this conclusion applies no less to those relatively rare unfortunates whose pattern of behaviour, inherited and reactive, is incompatible with the social order to a degree amounting to delinquency or criminality, sexual and otherwise. Although in the light of scientific insight, it is inappropriate to blame or punish, it is equally inappropriate that society or any individual members thereof should be exposed to injury at their hands, either before or after terms of punitive imprisonment. Through our lack of understanding and through our own emotional reactions we make both mistakes. What is more important than the inappropriate blamings and punishings, is our failure to appreciate that indi-viduals with such behaviour-patterns will continue compulsively to repeat them at the expense of a society that has been foolish enough to give them renewed opportunity.

In this connection it occurs to me to say that the frustrations which society and economics place upon an early, full heterosexual, marital relationship are a most potent factor in encouraging these morbid products, or shall we say, in delaying or deferring full psychosexual maturity. Frustration puts a premium upon the development of component-instincts at the expense of mature sexual development and satisfactory personal relationships. Frustration, though designed to promote and encourage sublimation, and though perhaps to some extent successful in this respect, unfortunately has the effect of encouraging everything short of mature normal development. Frustration makes all perversions easier, including the tendency to repress them, but does not make full relationships an actual possibility until the individual has gone through such a long period of frustration that he may have lost the potentiality for a really desirable level of adaptation. Thus, social frustration, economic frustration, though promoting sublimations which maintain civilization, also promotes perversions, the repression of perversions, consequent neurosis, and the disturbance and impoverishn.ent of personal relationships.

CHAPTER XXV

WOMEN

THEORETICAL INTRODUCTION

MATTER behaves in accordance with its natural properties as shown by the laws of chemistry and physics, and this incontrovertible rule applies to animate matter no less than to inanimate. In the course of evolution certain patterns of behaviour become elaborated physiologically and, later, psychologically, and passed on by the process of growth and reproduction.

The biogenic basis of human relationship, as indeed of all psychological action and reaction, is of course, instinct. Inherited patterns of behaviour, or instincts, as they are called, have been said by psycho-analysts to be of two principal varieties, the libidinal and the destructive, sometimes called the life instinct and the death instinct. The clinical, practical or actual aspects of these are held to be the pleasure-giving instinct, and the aggressive or destructive instinct. The latter is most commonly observed as reactive, as though it were mobilised for the purpose of removing obstacles in the path of our pleasure.

Perhaps we need not go into the other tenets of psycho-analysis in connection with the so-called death instinct, except to mention that it includes such clinical phenomena as repetition (sometimes called repetitive instinct), and the idea that it can be turned inwards and cause internal destruction. There is the further, perhaps philosophical, idea that it is responsible for, or has something to do with, our ultimate decease.

Be all that as it may, most analysts have accepted the idea of there being two very basic instincts, namely one which makes for pleasure or the removal of discomfort, and the other which is characterized more by aggressive and destructive tendencies. Now I would say that our personal relationships are based on these biogenic patterns or instincts, *plus* something else. This something else, next only to the primitive or inherited basis in importance, is, in my opinion, elaborations, alterations, modifications, and denials of these basic instinctual reactions, which have come about during our very early babyhood, childhood, and infancy. Although the latest psycho-analytical tendency is to concentrate attention upon the first weeks and months of the baby's relationship to the breast or bottle, believing that subsequent relationships follow the first-established pattern, it is said that object-relationship in the fullest sense is only finally established at what is called the Oedipus level, the level of full genital organisation. This is said to be the level of emotional development at which the infant first becomes capable of a full *whole*-object relationship in the sense of a person as such.

Therefore, it may be said that the psychology of our human relationships is based upon, one, the biologically inherited emotional patterns or instincts, libidinal and destructive, and, two, elaborations and modifications superimposed upon these instinctual bases and brought about specifically at the Oedipus level of emotional development, in relationship to parents or parents-surrogate.

After all, this idea is not so very surprising when we remember that the first experience of a personal relationship that any individual has is, as an infant, becoming cognizant of the people around him, particularly of his mother and father, and their specific natures and qualities, and being aware of certain reactions within him specifically to these particular individuals. Throughout his life thereafter he will meet individuals and will naturally react to them on the basis of his earliest acquired reactions, those reactions acquired at such an early and malleable stage of development that they produce and establish changes in his reactive pattern.

Thus, we have, in the reactive pattern, acquired if not inherited, at the Oedipus level of development, what might be called the infant-parent relationship. In other words, a reactive pattern is produced, acquired if not inherited (perhaps a bit of both), in the child during its very early stages of development; and it is the reactive pattern of the infant towards his parents and towards other adults. This reactive pattern, like all others acquired in earliest life, remains throughout the individual's existence. Some may hold that this is something quite distinct from the sexual pattern, but there is a great deal of analytical clinical evidence to indicate that it is not so different. It *appears* to be different. Soon after birth the infant reacts to its mother with a sensual, physical lust, differing from that of an adult chiefly in that its organ is the mouth and its function sucking. It may be remembered that these tendencies remain associated with subsequent sexual development. The biogenic instincts, libidinal and aggressive, inherited from the parents, undergo certain modifications during the course of the infant's development, or, rather, they acquire certain more elaborate patterns, in consequence of experience during infancy.

However, we can leave this subject, and merely remark that throughout the person's life a certain tendency to react as an infant to other persons and adults is natural in consequence, perhaps, of the years-long experience and development of this infant-parent reactive pattern during infancy and childhood. Psycho-analysts have no doubt that it is based upon the pleasure-pain (or gratification) principle and that it has a similar basis to what subsequently becomes recognizable as sexuality.

Then, there is, of course, the parent-infant reaction, something which grows with one it seems, and is characteristic of the good mother. Whether such a reactive pattern can be regarded as having been developed in infancy may be questioned, but the fact remains that it is there or shows itself if the person achieves full emotional maturity, and, particularly, if she becomes a parent. It is conceivable, or rather it is in line with analytical experience, that even this pattern, or its particular variations, might have been acquired in infancy, for, although the infant is reacting in what I have called the infant-parent pattern of reaction, nevertheless there are two persons involved, the parent as well as the infant, and it only needs the individual to identify himself with the other party in the relationship to have some experience or feeling of the parent-infant reactive pattern.

I have come across much analytical evidence to show that where there is a reciprocal reaction between two persons the child or infant can easily acquire an aptitude for both patterns. It is as though you saw a play with only two characters in it time and time again, repeated year in year out, and although you yourself played one of the roles, the infant role, nevertheless you got to know the other role as played by the other actor, the parent, so thoroughly that it was only a short step to play their part for them under certain circumstances.

The patient I mentioned once before, who was brought up by a very severe and strict stepmother, seemed to show throughout

his life two patterns of reaction to persons around him: Either he
was the infant, a little boy, helpless and fearful, full of the anxieties
which he had experienced as a child, or—this was the astonishing
thing—he could almost equally, with equal facility, become the
great tyrant, just like his stepmother. Indeed, when he was
reacting that way, he even spoke with a voice similar to hers.
Such evidence supports the idea that tyranny breeds tyranny, and
kindness breeds kindness.

Well, now we have postulated three reactive patterns, one, the
inherited, sexual and aggressive, an instinctual pattern; two, the
infant-parent reactive pattern; and, three, the parent-infant reactive
pattern. There are, no doubt, many others. One could suggest,
for example, a brotherly or sisterly reactive pattern, perhaps also
acquired during infancy and childhood in relation to siblings, to
brothers and sisters or other children with whom we have had
some emotional dealings during our babyhood and childhood.
Such patterns may include a sort of identification, brotherly or
sisterly love, and they can include also jealousy, fear, hatred,
murderous impulses, and even apathy.

The point I wish to stress is that, in addition to inherited
patterns, whatever reactive patterns we acquire in our malleable
period of life, during babyhood, infancy and childhood, we tend to
react to other persons throughout our lives in accordance with
these same inherited and acquired reactive patterns. Naturally,
it depends to some extent on which particular reactive pattern the
particular person stimulates. Some persons will stimulate our love
pattern, others our hate, but our reaction is not so completely
dependent on the real nature of the other person (certainly it is
not created by the other person), as it is a sort of repetition of a
pattern already laid down within us. For instance, some people
will hate even angels, and others will love even devils. Some are
imbued with fear—fear of almost everybody. Some are full of
pleasurable excitement and anticipation; others would appear to
be fed-up and apathetic. All these reactions, to whatever persons,
have their foundation not only in our inherited instincts but also
in the reactive patterns which we have acquired and developed
during our babyhood, infancy and childhood.

The compulsion to react in accordance with these patterns,
appropriately or often inappropriately, depends to some extent

upon the presence or absence of conflict, or rather upon the degree of conflict—as we all have conflict—and upon its nature. For instance, there are persons who seem to have a super-abundance of super-ego. They are liable to have a repressive and chilling effect on any person with whom they have any relationship. They have repressed their own libidinal and perhaps other emotional impulses—very often the libidinal more than the aggressive—and they tend to have a similar repressive effect upon ours, perhaps by reinforcing or stimulating our own equivalent tendencies, our own super-ego repressive tendencies. Our ability to react appropriately to a person, and indeed to any situation or stimulus, depends much more than is generally recognized, upon the pressure of the forces within us demanding outlet or relief. Every person's ego, reason as well as power of control, is more or less vitiated by the strength and urgency of his repressed instincts and complexes. Our reactions in a personal relationship and our capacity for appropriate thought and behaviour are much more limited than we imagine.

My professional experience convinces me that the last thing any of us wants to do, despite protestations to the contrary, is to change, or to modify in the slightest degree, our accustomed reactive patterns. They have become part of us, identified with ourselves, with our pleasure life, and anyone who tries to interfere with them is our enemy or executioner. What we are all keen about is to modify, not ourselves, but our environment and those around us, so that we can go on comfortably reacting in our customary way unchecked.

CHAPTER XXVI

INHIBITED WOMEN

IN these chapters I have, perhaps rather arbitrarily, followed a scale corresponding to the degree of libidinal or sexual freedom displayed by a succession of patients. I have adopted this scale because this is a matter (instinct level if you like, or rather instinct modified by the reactive pattern superimposed upon it) which has one of the greatest of all effects upon personal relationships, whether at first, second, third or any other interview. I have mentioned in previous chapters how I received some male patients who appeared to have succeeded in repressing their sexuality to an incredible degree. Well, naturally, the same applies in the case of females.

First I shall take a case of a young woman who was brought to see me because she was rather depressed. When I say 'young' . . . well, she looked extraordinarily young. I was not the only one who thought so, for she had been much offended, she told me, on several occasions when, going out with a party to a saloon bar or Club, she had been informed by the manager that girls under eighteen were not admitted. Yet, believe it or not, her age at that time was no less than twenty-eight. She was twenty-eight, but could easily have passed for a schoolgirl. It occurred to me that there must have been some retardation of her emotional development to keep her looking so young. There was no mental defect, as measured by ordinary standards, for this young lady actually had a university degree; and here she was, at the age of twenty-eight, brought to a psychologist because she was suffering from depression.

At her interview one of the first things she said to me was that her chief trouble was that she would like to get married, and in spite of wishing so much to get married no young man had actually come her way. Not knowing her at all well, just looking at her at the first interview, this seemed rather amazing because she was one of the sweetest and prettiest girls I had ever seen. What is more she had just expressed her conscious wish to get married. One might have thought that her difficulty would be how to keep the men away, how to keep out of marriage. But no, no man had ever come into her life. Had she lived in a jungle all the time? Whatever could be the explanation of this? Certainly she was very quiet, and modest and retiring, but one might have thought that this would make her all the more attractive.

Then she told me a little story of something that had happened a short time previously, a story which seemed to explain a good deal, if not everything, about the situation. One of her brothers was connected with the Navy, and there had been a dance on some battleship. One of the ship's officers, a particularly nice young man, had invited her to accompany him on to the boat deck in the moonlight, where so many other couples had gone between dances. No sooner had she got up there with him than some extraordinary fear overcame her. He had not made the slightest advance, had always been the soul of politeness, said nothing even suggestive that the situation between him and her was anything but formal and polite. Nevertheless, the situation caused her to feel an extraordinary fear. She said: 'I felt something in my stomach, in the whole of my stomach, as though all my inside were being tightened up, and drawn into my chest.' Evidently, drawn away from the man, into a position tucked away securely under her diaphragm! She said: 'It was as though everything were tied up in a great knot and drawn in towards me. It was an awful feeling; I felt somehow terrified, panic-stricken. We had hardly been up there a few minutes when I said to him, "I must go down, I must go down at once." He seemed surprised, but he escorted me from the boat deck down the steps that we had, the moment before, gone up.'

This little story seemed to me to explain a great deal. Her reaction to the male, to the, shall we say, biologically sound situation of the presence of a potential mate, was not that of libidinal feeling, pleasure, anticipation; it was just one great fear—an anticipation, not of pleasure, but of disaster, or something terrible. For this reaction to supervene she did not have to wait until some advance or love approach was made—no, the very atmosphere of the possibility of such a thing was enough. Thus, one could see that, although on a conscious level she said, 'I want a man, I want marriage', the truth of the matter was that she was panic-stricken even at the possibility of such a thing arising. Emotionally, fundamentally, she was not looking for a man, she was not looking for a mate, she was taking every precaution to flee from one. That is why she was not married. She was in flight, in panic-stricken flight, almost before the man's shadow appeared on the horizon.

An explanation of this was not hard to seek. Emotionally she was but a little girl, a little girl of six or seven, but of course a little girl with intelligent ideas and a knowledge of things sufficient to make her believe that she ought to get married. After all, she was now twenty-eight—though emotionally more like eight. It was not that this girl had no sexual life—something was going on, but it was in no wise connected with reality. It had no relationship to any real man, or to anything real. What went on was purely a phantasy, and to a large extent, I think, a subconscious phantasy.

In the course of analysis gradually it came out. There was a sort of saga, a romantic saga, more than romantic, a biological saga. It makes me think of *The Forsyte Saga*. In the saga she married some cousin of hers, and had children, and the children married, and they had children, and their children married, and they had children, and so the generations went on and developed and multiplied; all was very beautiful and loving and romantic. Like one of Guyon's 'uterine type' of woman, with no vestige of 'clitorid' character, she was not consciously aware of genital sensation, although there were phantasies of reproduction, nursing and growing up of babies, and so on. The one baby that never seemed to grow up was herself.

Well, in the course of analysis this 'child' of twenty-eight went through certain stages of development which normally would have occurred perhaps fifteen years earlier. In due course she masturbated, and had conflict about it, and certain phantasies about it, and certain fears about it, just like any girl at puberty or adolescence. She had phantasies about men, certain men she had met in the past, and did meet in the present. But, I am afraid that the reality contact was very, very slow in developing. Her Oedipus fixation was very firm indeed. Oedipus fixation means, of course, that one loves the father, is married to the father, but, naturally, father has no genitals. The other side of it is where there are genitals; where there is overt sexuality, of course there is no father. Genitality becomes a sort of perversion, which is wrong, wicked, and full of worry and conflict. Father-fixation and sexuality are, as it were, divorced, split, from each other. (What a lot of this nonsense still exists in our bringing up of children and in our half-baked society of to-day!)

Nevertheless, her sexuality did develop. She had a wonderful phantasy—almost more than a phantasy; it actually became a 'plan'. She said an institution ought to be established in which women like herself would go in at one end and be vetted by doctors; men would go in at another door and be similarly vetted. Each would then go through a sort of changing house in which each would be clad in a black garment that blotted out all the face and all the body, and left exposed only the genitals. Then, under proper medical auspices, a male and a female would be put together, and sexuality would take place with satisfaction. Then they would be separated and the doctors and nurses would revet them, and reclothe them. The whole thing would be a sort of authentic medical, surgical—or gynaecological—treatment. This phantasy was a way of getting the sexual instinct gratified with complete security, and without having to make personality adjustments in connection with it.

This woman's personality adjustments were, of course, characterized by great timidity, or rather, so far as possible by avoidance. As on the boat deck with the young man, she was in retreat. The pattern had been so long established—right up to the age of twenty-eight—that she was difficult from every point of view. Nevertheless, slowly but surely, development did take place. Her periods became regular, and her sexuality might be said to have come within the limits of normality, though I would prefer to say it reached the limit that was *for her* consistent with her greatest happiness and least anxiety.

I now think of another sex-inhibited young woman of similar age. She was the perpetual school-girl, student or undergraduate. She had gone through one course of training after another. The reason was that, having been trained and qualified, in some particular line—first of all, it was domestic science and cooking—she hardly felt adult enough to put it to any practical use. Children and adolescents can be trained, but they can hardly be expected to take on a responsible job and do work and earn a living. So, after years of domestic-science training, she then adopted another training.

This time it was physiotherapy. She went through three years of that, and got fully qualified. That was the stage at which she came to me. The reason was that she could not work, she could not *do* physiotherapy, however well she had been trained. She did try. In the early stages of her analysis she tried. She got a job in a hospital, and was doing some electrical treatment on a patient when she saw the doctor, or some male, come in at the far end of the ward. She immediately fled through the furthermost door.

Finally, she took a third training, which I had better not mention in case of revealing her identity, and there, eventually, she did very well indeed. All this happened a great time ago. She got a job, a responsible and important job, and she worked at it for ten years. At the end of ten years of hard work, very useful work, she came to me. She had visited me a few times in the interim period, but at the end of ten years she came to me, and she said: 'My parents are rich. Shall I give up this work and retire home? Of course, I know what will happen. Mother will get me into her clutches again. But, after all, I have done what you told me to do, I have done ten years, every day from nine o'clock to five, apart from holidays, vacations, and very rare illnesses. Do you think I should stop it now?'

I looked at her and thought to myself, 'Have I, I, the psychologist, done the right thing?' I had, as it were, pushed this poor girl into this hard-working job. Admittedly it was very much the same sort of job that most people do, without ever thinking that they are undergoing any special strain. What is the difference between them and this girl? The difference is this: that this poor creature was a neurotic. She was really immature and emotionally under-developed, though not so under-developed as when she first came. Nevertheless she was a neurotic and under-developed. She had been on her toes for ten years, with nervous strain all the time. I thought: this has been a bit of a cruelty, I should not have let her do it. I should have encouraged her to resign the job long ago. It should have been enough for her to prove to herself that she *could* do it; but *ten* years!—good gracious, this cruelty has gone on too long. I took my cue from her questions, and said: 'Of course, you've done it quite long enough. Give it up now.' One might have added, 'Be yourself. Have your neurosis,' for that would be less of a hardship, less of a torture than trying to be normal like this.

Now, what was conspicuously immature in this girl, as in the first, was the matter of sexual development. She had wonderful phantasies of going to hospitals and to doctors, and being physically examined, and getting a terrific thrill out of it. She was more advanced than the previous case, however, because she did have quite definite and almost real, practical ideas of courtship and lovemaking, and had, now I come to think of it, had a few minor experiences in that direction. But, and this was her safeguard, she was terribly fussy about whom it should be that she should marry. For one thing, it had to be a doctor. For another, he had to be a certain age, for another, he had to be a bachelor, for another, he had to have had no previous sexual experience. All these stipulations made her pretty safe against having to surrender herself to a mate. Her sexual life was confined to rather less mature phantasies than these.

I cannot tell you what an extraordinary primitive sexual or erotic level she was on when she first came to me. However, I may say this: although she was then thirty, she had not at that time discovered that she had a genital organ. Her personal relationships, like those of the previous case, were more like the personal relationships one would expect from a small child, although this 'child' was a little older than the previous one. I should say she was more like fourteen or fifteen than seven or eight. Her chief erotic pleasure at that time, at that stage of her life, at the age of thirty, was enemas.

CHAPTER XXVII

THE SOCIALITE

PERSONAL RELATIONSHIP IN LIEU OF SEXUAL RELATIONSHIP

PROCEEDING from very morbid states of sex repression to those a little less extreme, and perhaps more familiar, I think now of a woman who was almost a socialite. She shone in society. If not the soul of the party, she was something very near it. She was most agreeable to meet, her conversation held one emotionally and everybody liked her. What was wrong with her personal relationships? Surely, these were very mature, or even ideal. Well, I will tell you what was wrong with them: They *were* her sexuality—not a part of it, but the whole of it. She enjoyed social relationships; what she could not enjoy was her husband getting into bed with her. That was what she could not enjoy. I think her sexuality was going on all the time she was socially mixing with people; if anything became more intimate than that, it stopped.

Now this woman had divorced her first husband, and recently, at the age of nearly forty, married a second. It was within six months of this second marriage that she came to see me. She explained that her first husband had really been impossible; they had practically not lived together. Then, once upon a time, travelling abroad, she had met this second husband. He was a married man in the middle forties, but he had fallen so much in love with her, her cheerful, gay social disposition, that he had decided then and there that he must be quit of his wife, and marry this one. She had not been to the same extent enamoured of him. In fact, she said to me: 'What an extraordinarily selfish man he must have been! Always trying to press marriage on me, without any consideration for what *I* felt about marrying him. He took no regard for *my* feelings. He was concerned only with his own.'

At one time he had in fact been so unfeeling as to think that she would do very well as the other-woman-in-the-case, to enable him to divorce his wife. With this plan in view, he had on holiday obtained a suite for them to share together in a big hotel. They arrived at their hotel, and he escorted her into a room with a double bed in it. She took one look at him at the double bed, and at the programme, and burst into tears. Mind you, this was a woman of nearly forty. She thought it was all horrid. She nearly finished with him on the spot. Nothing happened for many months, but after she had divorced her husband, and this man's freedom was imminent, she went on an innocent platonic holiday with him. She went on to tell me that, during this holiday, on one occasion, this man of hers actually raped her. Nevertheless, some twelve or eighteen months later, her resistances had been borne down, and finally she married him.

Then again, she said to me: 'Do you know, on the bridal night, this horrible fellow was bad enough to do the same thing again. He raped me for the second time.'

Now this woman's history of herself and her life, the stories she told—particularly the way she told them—were very entertaining and in an unsophisticated way fascinating. They were like a good novel, interestingly coloured by her character and personality. The reason she had come to see me was that this marriage, like the first one, was proving quite impossible. Right from the start, it was quite impossible. Admittedly, she had been earning her own living most of her unmarried life, and, admittedly, this second husband was quite well off. He had a good business and brought in a good income. She was given a liberal housekeeping allowance and a joint banking account; but all these material advantages weighed as nothing with her. It was the personality of the man that was impossible. He was dull, stupid, uninteresting.

I got the impression that the fact of the matter was that he was normal sexually, and she was not. I saw too that she had a tremendous capacity for transference—she was getting it towards me—a tremendous capacity for transference—providing nothing physically intimate happened—no 'rape'. Sociability was her sexuality. I foresaw some real practical difficulties ahead. Here she was, a woman of nearly forty, proposing to divorce the husband she had been married to for little over six months. She had no independent income, no funds. All she could have done would have been to start a job, similar to the one she had had earlier in her life, on about seven pounds a week. And, frankly, I could not see her living on it.

Here, I hinted at a very extraordinary and unusual course. I think I knew when I hinted at it, that it could not possibly succeed. It was the matter of putting one's backing on reality, as against emotion. I said to her: 'You have been a very hard-working girl in your time. You've worked from nine a.m. to five p.m. How many hours is that? Well, how many hours do you see your husband; I understand he's out early in the morning at his factory, and back home not until six or seven o'clock at night, and you both go to bed at about half past eleven. You have a separate room—you sleep separately in separate rooms. Do you think it would be possible to make your marriage to this man, who doesn't seem to have any very great or impossible peculiarity—he's normal enough in most respects, and potent—don't you think you might be able to make your marriage to him a sort of "job"? Just keep him happy, and see how things work that way?'

She looked at me steadily, and took it all in. But knowing what little I already knew about her, I fancied that her capacity to make her emotions, her emotional life, secondary to her reality sense, was practically non-existent. And actually, I may as well confess it, I wanted to get rid of this patient. I could see no solution to the situation, and I did not want to be involved in it. I could see that she would get an increasingly strong transference to me, and that she would, by hook or by crook, divorce her husband and have no money. By that time, I imagined she would be so attached to me and to my treatment, that it would be a cruelty to try and get rid of her. That, perhaps, is why I thought: 'We'll see what she can do if we give her a chance on this "job" idea. At any rate, at the job of marriage to this man, she would "earn", in a sense, perhaps nearly a hundred times what she would have been earning on her own account.' It weighed absolutely nothing with her.

I think it was at her very next session she said to me: 'All last week I was still trying to follow your suggestion of making a "job" of the marriage. Well, I'm afraid I can't do it. The misery, the dullness and the boredom—even if it's only a little time we spend together! I cannot bear it. The pattern has been established, and I can't stand the pattern. Last night we had another of our flaming rows. I'm afraid that, far from doing my "job", I was the one who brought it about—as usual. We had been sitting together in the lounge for a little time, and I started the row. It was because I couldn't sit in that room any longer. It was only about nine p.m., and I said: "I'm going to my room." Everything had been silent and peaceful up to that moment. He said, looking up from his newspaper, "Why, it's only nine o'clock."

'I said: "I'm decidedly bored." Yes, I know I was not doing my "job", as you told me to.'

'Well, what had happened that made you say this to him?'

She said: 'Nothing, absolutely nothing. You can enjoy sitting with somebody if there is a rapport between you, but sitting with my husband like this! I knew it was a silence born out of nothing to say. I think I started the row just to have a little excitement. Well, that was not necessarily conscious. I suppose I expected some kind of reaction when I said, "I'm bored." His first reaction was very calm. I said to him: "We can't go out every evening, I know, but when we are at home together, I find it just impossible." By this time I had aroused him a bit too, and he said: "I find you dull also." I said: "I want to do something about it." He said: "You can't do anything with me. It's the way I am."

'I said: "I was naïve enough to think that you wanted to be changed. I will have to recognize that you will not change."

'Then he said: "Perhaps I could change, if you would help me." Then he went on, after I had provoked him a bit further, to a list of complaints about me as a wife. He reached the question of our sexual relationship which, I admit, is very bad. He said that I wouldn't be different with any man, that I simply don't care about sex. Well, what if that were true? Can't two people get on without sex? Yes, it was a row. At times we were angry. He said there was no point in going on, that he was leaving then and there because I didn't care a damn about him. The row went on for hours and hours. In the early morning I went to my room. I was in a terrible state. I had to take my usual sleeping pills, and a bit more.

'He had said to me that I have a good life, and am not contented because I demand far too much. I said to him: "You mean, you provide material comfort." Presently he accused me of being too intellectual. I replied, that I expected something more than material comfort; I expected some kind of companionship. I was not doing all this rowing deliberately. I was thinking of future evenings; no conversation unless I make it. He has nothing to say, no views, no ideas, nothing. He asked me what I found so wrong with him. I said, "You don't think." He said: "How does one go about thinking?" How should he learn to think? What fooled me into marrying this man was that he convinced me that he really wanted to co-operate. Then, I find that all he wants is—well, goodness knows what—sex, anyway. Oh, yes, he's potent all right. I wish he wasn't. I get nothing out of it.'

One might sum-up this patient's psychopathology by saying that she fails to get adequate psychosexual satisfaction in intercourse. She gets more gratification out of non-physical emotional relationships; for instance, in society, and that is why I felt she would get·a very strong transference to me if I let her treatment continue. Because she gets no satisfaction out of physical relationships, she feels repugnance for the man, and therefore, for all his personal ways and habits, even to his sitting in the room with her; and that is why she rows.

If she controls her emotional expression, for instance, if she suppresses her tendency to row, she gets psychosomatic or hysterical symptoms, pains in her side, and migraine. She is an hysteric, unsuited, in my opinion, for any man, and suited only for transference, that is for psychotherapy; or for some social, superficial, emotional relationships to people, relationships that do not include anything physical.

I felt that this woman could not, in her present state, succeed in sexual adjustment to a man on account of the hysterical nature of her emotional life. In other words, my impression was that 'sex' was going on in all her ordinary relationships, but it was sex in phantasy. That is why her social life was so stimulating, and that is why she was so stimulating socially. Sex goes on in phantasy only, and is stimulated by personal relationships and personal contacts. One could feel it even in a first interview with her. But her sexuality is stopped by any real physical approach, particularly of course, by anything like sexual intercourse. This is almost certainly because of some unconscious father fixation.

To sum up, one might say that her capacity for transference is infinitely greater than her capacity for sexual love or for marriage. She was so addicted to her neurosis, to her hysteria, to her emotional life, and her need to live it in accordance with its pattern that otherwise she would be ill. Here, I felt she was correcting my, perhaps stupid, advice that she should make a 'job' of her marriage, because if she does not deal with her neurosis by the device of living socially and asexually, she is ill. Therefore, I felt, perhaps the patient was more sensible than I was. Anyhow, be that as it may, here was a woman who was determined to take her own 'advice', that is to say to gratify her emotional pattern, to express it anyway, whether she would gratify it or not, to live in accordance with her emotional need, irrespective of reality if reality conflicted with that need. So I could see nothing but disaster ahead. I said to her, 'Well, all right, if you must get rid of your husband, what will you do then? You've told me that you will go back to work, work at seven or eight pounds a week, after the way you. have been accustomed to living. How will that agree with you? I can't see you living on that income.'

She said: 'Well, Doctor, would you advise me to get married again?'

I looked at her, and thought to myself, 'What an inflated idea this woman must have of herself! Here, she is, a confirmed hysteric, quite useless to any man in a mating or married relationship, a socially-adjusted but not a sexually-adjusted infant, and yet she is asking me if she should get married again! I can't conceive of any man being fool enough to want to marry such a bad bargain, the worst bargain in wives that I have ever met.' I said to her: 'Why do you ask me? Have you anything in view?'

'Well,' she said to me, 'Yes, I have! The only trouble is that I am not very much in love with the man, just as it was with this husband. He's quite all right, and all that, but I cannot say that I am really in love with him at all. He is with me, and very much wants to marry me.'

Then it transpired that there were also no less than two others! Well, well, this was a matter that gave one some food for thought. How was it that the least desirable of all women as a wife, when one knew and understood her psychopathology, had men lined up, even when she was forty years of age and twice divorced, pressing to marry her? What was the explanation of this? Perhaps the explanation of it was that her social life, her personal contacts, were so imbued with emotion, so stimulating and pleasing, that the male subconsciously assumed that sexuality with her would be equally, or similarly, or more, pleasing and interesting and en-joyable in every way. Of course the truth is, he did not think at all, he just got a blind transference to her.

Another possibility that occurred to me, perhaps not contradictory to this one, was this: In view of her husband's so-called rapings of her, perhaps he himself was sexually immature enough to have an element of sadism in him, and want to force himself upon an unwilling victim, on something emotionally comparable to a child of eight, nine or ten. Naturally such a concept would certainly be repressed by his super-ego and ego. However, when he sees a woman of forty with that degree of emotional immaturity, there he can enjoy his particular form of 'perversion'.

However true or untrue this may be, I certainly think that there is another element, and that is that this socially, one might almost say, brilliant, woman, had something of the quality of a mother-image about her. It seems to be a contradiction to say that she was a child and in the same breath to say that she had a mother characteristic about her. Perhaps one might say that she was a child sexually, when it came to intercourse or physical intimacy, but a mother socially. Thus, the symptomatic behaviour on the part of her husband, of pressing for her hand in marriage might be over-determined in at least two respects: one, that his undeveloped component-instinct of sadism was attracted from the point of view of shall we call it, 'rape', and the other determinant would be, two, that his mother-fixation—very often related to such a degree of psychological undevelopment—that his mother-fixation-element felt that here was lovely mother that he could have in his own possession for ever. Well, we know what he got, and we may hazard a rough guess as to what any future husband will get.

CHAPTER XXVIII

FRIGIDITY AND ORGASTIC FRIGIDITY

IT was in the early years of the last world war that a young woman came clattering into my consulting room with a tin hat, gas mask, and a whole lot of paraphernalia and equipment. A greater misrepresentation of her real psychology could hardly be imagined, except for the fact that emotionally she was something of a tomboy, a sort of adolescent or boyish male. At this first interview she was so pleasant and taking, as chatty and intelligent as the bright boy of the class, that one might be excused for wondering why she had come to consult me; and yet this was one of the most intractable cases of nervous illness that I have encountered. There was nothing wrong with her intelligence; she was all right at the ego level. The trouble, as usual, lay more deep-seatedly, down at the emotional and unconscious level.

She mixed with all sorts and conditions of people, apparently quite happily, males and females of every age and station. She rather preferred the humbler classes to people of any social position. Nevertheless, she appeared to be happy, if a little intense, with all and sundry. We shall see that all this was largely a cover. Deep down she *felt* the truth: It was that she had never developed into a *woman*. She was still a child, a boy, a *gamin*.

In due course it transpired that the idea of a male-friend, in the sense of a prospective or possible mate, had never so much as entered her head, although she was now nearly thirty. She was a slim, boyish little person, and might easily have passed for twenty. Her emotional retardation, or lack of development, extended far deeper than this absence of any desire for a mate. She did need somebody; she needed a man, a big, strong, middle-aged or elderly man; but what she needed him for was one thing, and one thing only. She longed to be cuddled by him! Not to be cuddled in the ordinary passionate or sexual manner, but quite specifically to be what she called, 'held tight'. She wanted to be held tight, *and that was all she wanted*. She wanted to be held tight all her life. The reason was that, otherwise, the world was peopled with all kinds of terrors and dangers of an indescribable nature. One might call them 'bogies'. She lay awake through the nights fearful, fearing. The one thing she felt that could dispel her anxiety was this great, big, strong father-figure. Sex meant less than a little to her, it meant nothing. In fact, it meant so little that she was not averse to experimenting with it. It seemed she did not even mind a little bit of sexual intercourse now and again, provided—and this was the important part of it—that the man was a father-figure, and that he held her tight. If she could not induce him to hold her tight by any other means, well then . . . well, that did not matter very much. In any case, it was quite meaningless to her, certainly quite meaningless sexually. She was totally and absolutely frigid.

She was more gravely ill than these things indicated. Her inheritance, from a psychopathological point of view, from both parents, was very bad. Several of her close relatives had ended their life by suicide, but here she was, at this interview with me, apparently normal, and, well, happier than most people.

Later on she told me that she *was* happy at this interview. No sooner had she come in and seen me, a man of the age that mattered from the point of view of the relief of her anxieties, and found me kindly and disposed to listen to her, than she was immediately quite well! The trouble or difficulty about conveying her condition to me was that, with me, in my presence, she had no condition. All was well so long as she was with me. But what a different story in the nights when she lay in her bed alone, when all the bogies were around her, and no kind 'father' present!

To cut a long story short, one can say with confidence that this woman's personal relationships were based upon an infant-kind-father emotional pattern. As a very small infant, she had been left at four years of age, when her mother had died—apparently by an accident. She had been left in the sole care of her father. Now, the father was a highly neurotic, eccentric, and altogether very odd man. He was subject to occasional spasms of hysterical affection—when he would grab a child and squeeze it passionately—alternating with fits of unreasonable temper. He had beaten the small children quite a lot. But the worst thing he did to this child apparently was when he sent her to a boarding school. She realized from that moment that she was not wanted, not wanted by anyone. And then she saved herself by nursing the idea that after all, father *did* want her. At the end of term, father would come for her. She would be in father's arms, and, lo and behold, all security in life and all happiness would be restored. Tragedy followed; for, when she was with father eventually, at the end of term, he took little or no notice of her—unless by some accident or other she came under his ill graces, or fell into his clutches when he was in a temper. Then he beat her. But the phantasy she nursed during term-time, of a good father, remained. Apparently it operated as soon as she came into my consulting room, and that is why she was so well, and gave me such a wrong impression of herself.

However, for our purposes the point is that this girl's relationships to people varied according to whether or not they could be put in the category of the 'good father' whom she had sought throughout her childhood and infancy. If they could be put into that category, all was perfect; it was a lovely world, and she was happy. If they could not be put into that category, well, she was apathetic as far as they were concerned. There was no emotional rapport, no personal relationship. She was left with her bogies. Or, worse than this, in some people's company, quite frequently things might be on the side of the bogies; they might be bad people, dangerous; and her anxiety state would be increased in their presence instead of lessened. She was quite hopeless with them, and yet quite helpless; very often even helpless enough not to be able to get away; but get away she did, sooner or later. She could not live in a boarding house or hotel on account of these things. She led a very lonely and solitary life, hoping always for the good father. She said to me, at a later date: 'When I came to you . . . well, just coming to you, I was cured. I was all right so long as I kept coming.'

She had a course of analysis, and naturally all her hatred for her father became projected on to me in due course, and her symptoms returned. But her transference had sufficient positive elements in it to save her from tragedy, and to restore her to a modicum of good health, and to an ability to earn a good living.

Now this patient was obviously in the category of those with deficient sexual development; and, connected with this, her capacity for personal relationships, her rapport, was very limited and one-sided. It was confined to middle-aged or elderly men, and neurotic women, like herself, who told her of anxiety symptoms similar to those from which she suffered. Therefore she felt they 'understood'. She is now free from requiring these reassurances.

The next case I think of is one which gives the impression or appearance of having rather an excess of sexual development. She was a wife in the early thirties who was brought to me by her husband because, after barely ten years of marriage, she had started a passionate love affair with a man who was obviously an irresponsible and psychopathological type.

What may have given the impression that she was a bit over-sexed rather than under-sexed was the fact that, though she married her husband at twenty-two, she had previously had what seemed at first sight to be a fairly large number of affairs, during her bachelor days, and, what is more, these affairs practically all progressed to full sexual relationship. What might be still more striking is the fact that full sexual relationship commonly developed at her very first meeting with a man whom she fancied. These men were of all ages, a fair number of them being distinctly middle-aged. She was a pretty and attractive girl, with a slim figure. Men fell for her right and left, and if she fancied them, well, she just went to bed with them. Nothing else seemed to interest her. Indeed, it seemed that she could talk of little or nothing else. It was just going to bed with men, sleeping with them, sexual inter-course. That was what interested her, and that was what she talked about practically all the time.

Therefore, it was rather interesting, when we went further into the matter, to discover that this woman did not really experience any adequate sexual response. In fact, she got hardly any sexual response. She did get a little; it was quite pleasant to be having intercourse—well, like sucking a toffee. Never was there the slightest hint or vestige of anything really exciting, and certainly of nothing even approaching an orgasm.

Yes, she had masturbated quite a lot as a child. Her mastur-bations were all of them short of orgasm. When she reached puberty she was still masturbating, but in adolescence, with her first affair, it ceased. She took up with the boys, with sexual inter-course, in preference to masturbation. Why she preferred it, it is difficult to tell, as I am quite sure her account of her experiences during intercourse was correct. The thing was a very ordinary, simple, pleasurable sensation of a mild degree, and never produced anything like satisfaction.

This woman's personal relationships were definitely defective. She was introverted. She tended to withdraw into herself. At parties or at any social meeting I think everyone would find her cold and withdrawn, apparently apathetic, disinterested. The one asset from that point of view which she did have was her very attractive appearance; but when we have said appearance, we have said almost everything sexual about her.

The point about the new man, the new affair, which so disturbed her marital life, was the fact that this man could keep up sexual intercourse for an inordinate time. She did not get orgasm; he did not get orgasm, and, therefore, she thought he was wonderful. Her husband, on the other hand, was rather quick, and more interested in his business and ego-affairs than in sexuality. Nevertheless, she had remained faithful for all these nine or ten years of her married life. But, in the absence of these silly little affairs of hers, such as she had been having so frequently before she married, she became steadily more depressed. I fancy that the affairs were just straws at which she clutched in her depression, and that they too would have failed her in time.

If one had to classify this woman in a psychoneurotic or psychopathological category, one would classify her as a depressive-introvert, as being always introverted and subject to depression with recurrent exacerbations. Mostly she was apathetic—not only to sexual stimulation, but to people and personal contacts, and to everything; but not so apathetic as to give an impression of being abnormal. She was just deadly dull and uninteresting on every emotional plane. Nevertheless, she had a lot of good qualities, or at least the absence of bad ones. She did not have that super-ego-paranoid attitude to life—incidentally they often go together—which makes people feel guilty and miserable in the subject's presence. If she did not have much genuine stimulating and good effect upon people, she certainly did not have any bad effect either.

There was something to be said for her sexual attitude also, because the poor woman was nearly always dull and depressed if there were no men around her, but I think 'the man' was only an illusion-boosted placebo. I fancy that, like the schizophrenic, she was too introverted really to enjoy physical contact. Perhaps, a modicum of feeling or something would awaken if there was a man about who might become a sexual partner. So, whatever emotional life she did have, was connected with a need for contributions to her self-love, self-esteem or narcissism together with some anticipated genital stimulation, however mild. Her capacity for personal relationship, whether at a first interview or otherwise, was thus conditioned by factors, entirely immature and selfish, but which in other respects contrast somewhat with those of the previous case.

Is it due to the blindness of man, itself a product of conflict and repression that some immature and narcissistic people with no capacity for warmth or depth in their personal relationships, nevertheless get themselves mated or married before the mistake is discovered—by both parties to it?

However, to understand all is to 'forgive' all, or at least to avoid indulgence in the usual deprecatory and condemnatory criticisms of what are, after all, products of natural laws. It is not possible to 'understand all' about this lady without realising that she is fundamentally a little child who is afraid to give her transference in personal contacts and afraid to surrender to relief in sexual contacts. This fear shows itself as resistance in analytical treatment, and robs her of her birthright of health and happiness. The cause of its existence is that when she actually was a little child, and, like every little child, needed affectionate parents to give her some feeling of security and to stimulate affection in her, she was left insecure and wanting. Therefore, though the need is still in her somewhere, she is afraid to admit it even to herself; she is afraid of being hurt and abandoned all over again. Hers is, therefore, largely the coldness of fear. She is the principal sufferer. Her prevailing emotion, seemingly her only alternative to coldness and apathy, is that of insecurity feelings and anxiety identical with the emotional tone of her affection-less childhood.

CHAPTER XXIX

AN 'OVER-SEXED' WOMAN

I NOW come to the case of what would appear to be an over-sexed woman. If she were not a 'nymphomaniac', she was not all that far removed from one; but that was not what she complained of when she came to see me. She complained, quite truthfully, of all the symptoms associated with a most acute anxiety state. She was a buxom, plump, rosy, jolly-looking woman in the early thirties. At first sight she may well have given some people the impression that nothing whatsoever could possibly be the matter with her; and, yet, a great deal was the matter.

She began with her first and worst symptom, a sadly common one in obsessional neuroses. She said: 'Doctor, I am terribly afraid of going mad.' This is regarded by many psychiatrists and psychoanalysts as a very important and serious symptom. It is said that those who have this phobia have it on good grounds; but I could not feel that this was the case, at least not in this particular patient. She elaborated her statement: 'I am terribly afraid of silence. I think about my mind all day long. Also, I am afraid of losing my speech, and I'm afraid that I am going to faint. The last is quite recent. For six months I've had terrible panics, attacks of acute anxiety, palpitation of the heart, tremblings. My hands get damp and clammy. Then there are guilt complexes that worry me, terrible wrong things I used to do a few years ago. Now I don't see how I could have done those things. I must have been abnormal for a very long time to have done them.'

Certainly this woman was in an anxiety state, and I think, now, that, even without this recital of her symptoms, one may have been able to detect the fact on closer scrutiny. In contrast to the last case I have described, she was almost palpitating with excitement, emotion and anxiety. But it did not somehow all seem to be anxiety. There appeared to be a predominant intensity of feeling and emotion about her, as though something must happen or she would burst. I should say that she was tumescent all the time, perhaps on the verge of orgasm—orgasm that never arrived. To

G

my mind, and I later interpreted it thus for her, the fear of going mad was the fear of having orgasm, of something out-of-control happening. She might have put it differently, and said, 'If I can't get relief (if I can't get orgasm), then I shall burst or go mad.'

From a personal relationship point of view, this state of affairs was evidently sensed in some peculiar way by nearly all the men she met. She was a woman who could hardly walk down the street without being followed. If she got in a public vehicle, men came and sat close to her—hungry wolves looking for prey!—and when she got off, she would find herself followed. If she went into a restaurant some man would come and sit at the table opposite her. He would endeavour to introduce himself, get into conversation with her, and try and find out where she lived. Things of that sort went on all the time, and she complained in a helpless sort of way about them.

I could not avoid contrasting these factual stories of hers with the opposite sort of thing, which I hear from sexually inhibited people, such as the first cases in this series of chapters. These young women all told me how there were not any men. No man ever spoke to them. They could not achieve an acquaintanceship with anybody, and yet they wanted so badly to get married. This woman, on the other hand, was married, and had a family, and yet she could not get away from men; they followed her everywhere. Why was it? She was not as good-looking as the others. Was it her subconscious or something—something, not exactly visible, but intuitively sensed—the emotional state which she was trying to suppress and conceal? As she most aptly and shamefacedly complained: 'I am followed everywhere like a bitch on heat!'

As the story progressed—not so much at the first interview, but subsequently—it transpired that the males not only followed, but, very often, quite usually, they caught up on her in spite of herself. Sometimes it did not worry her, but very often she was in a sort of panic running away from it, and yet they caught up. When her husband had been away she had had such a succession of affairs it could hardly be believed. She was living with one man after another, and others were visiting her while the man she was living with was out of the house. She did not seek these things—at least, not consciously. She was a nice woman. They just came upon her; they overwhelmed her. They were going on all the time. But, in those days she was apparently well, so far as her nerves were concerned, so far as any of these symptoms she had just related to me were concerned. All her anxiety symptoms arrived subsequently. She traced the beginning of them as follows:

She said: 'The fear of becoming insane came upon me after my husband returned from service abroad. He told me that he had met another girl abroad. That was an awful shock to me. It seemed most peculiar for my husband, for I had always regarded him as the good, old-faithful type, and so he was. First of all, I was obsessed with worry about it, but then presently, curiously enough, I started to enjoy thinking about it. I thought about it day and night. It became my chief emotional excitement. It superceded all my own affairs, and all that business. My husband went away, presumably to elope with the other girl. Two months later he came back, and told me he had made a frightful mistake. He told me that he loved me, that it was only me whom he loved. Nevertheless, the odd thing is that I could not forget this other woman. All sorts of things began to happen. I began to break things; I began to have hysterical upheavals; I shouted, and did the most loathsome things; I knocked a glass out of his hand. And then, one evening in bed, I felt the blood rush into my head, and the awful thought came: I know I am going mad? I got out of bed. I started running around, and my heart beat terribly quickly. There had been no symptoms, such as I have been telling you, until that moment. I had always been a bit highly strung, but always strong. I had occasionally been frightened of things, but never like this.'

This patient also was orgastically frigid, except for occasional orgasms connected solely with clitoris masturbation. She had masturbated since the age of ten years. She claimed never to have had anything approaching adequate vaginal sensation. If ever she got any sexual excitement, it had to be by means of the clitoris. So it seems rather an extraordinary thing that she was so addicted to sexual intercourse, and also an extraordinary thing that males were so addicted to seeking sexual intercourse with her. She certainly corresponded to Guyon's 'clitorid-type' of woman in these respects. All her symptoms seemed to indicate that she was on the verge of some enormous explosion, an explosion which never took place.

There was one symptom in particular which pointed to this. It was as follows: she suffered from insomnia; but when she did go off to sleep, she would very commonly, as often as not, have a sort of nightmare. The only evidence of this nightmare was the report from her husband. She would suddenly sit bolt upright in bed, still apparently asleep, shouting at the top of her voice, 'I am dying. I am dying. I am dying.' She would repeat it over and over again, and then, very often, her husband would awaken her, as he was afraid she would rouse the neighbours. But, on a few occasions, 'I am dying, I am dying,' would lead finally to her shouting, 'I am dead.' With that she always flopped back into bed sound asleep, and remembered nothing whatsoever of the incident in the morning.

From her analysis I am convinced that 'I am dying' was the expression of a conflict which included, one, an approaching tendency to orgasm, and, two, an equally strong and determined resistance to it. Somewhere in her unconscious, orgasm was associated with death, in the same way that on the conscious level it was associated with 'going mad', 'losing control', or—as she sometimes put it—'losing my speech, thinking I am going to faint.' Naturally, she resisted this awful calamity to the last ditch. But occasionally during her sleep her resistance was unavailing, and something supervened in spite of it. That is when she would shout, 'I am dead', and fall back on the pillow sound asleep. This was the nearest she ever got to full orgastic relief.

There is a great deal more that I could say about this case, both from an hereditary point of view, and from every other point of view. Her mother also was a strong, powerful, emotional hysteric. But, my chief reason for mentioning the case is to conclude this chain or series of women, starting with the most asexual, or emotionally cold, and finishing with a good example of an apparently very strongly sexed and passionate woman—at least to judge by the number of men that kept following her and by the amount of sexuality in which she had indulged, or, rather, which she attracted and which was thrust upon her by all and sundry.

The value of the case from our point of view is that here was sexuality associated with a personal relationship that drew heterosexual males towards her. She somehow gave them a feeling that orgasm, her satisfaction and theirs, was very near, and that she was accessible. She attracted them sexually. Her presence seemed to arouse a sort of excitement, comparable to the excitement that was unrelieved within her.

Thus, here we have an instance where the emotional state within this woman, conscious and unconscious, arouses in the course of her personal relationships a similar state in those around her. Immediately there is some sort of personal contact of a mental nature, it proceeds, almost precipitately, towards the aim of the sexual instinct, namely orgasm, even if it does not quite achieve that aim. If this woman had wanted husbands, she could have had a dozen, in fact, many dozens. But, however many she had had, I do not think that she would ever have come to rest. She would always have needed more and more, simply because some unconscious inhibition prevented satisfaction or relief from one and all. And what a restless, uncomfortable state the poor woman was in all the time! Daily she was asking herself and everybody around her, the obsessional question: 'Am I going mad?'

The purpose of this record is not a compendious exposition of psychopathology, treatment and amelioration, but simply to adduce evidence to illustrate my thesis that sexual object-relationship, due to sexual urges and patterns, however compulsive and unconscious, can be a vital factor in personal relationship even at the first contact or interview.

PARTS III TO V: PRACTICE

PART FIVE

THE UNCONSCIOUS BASIS

CHAPTER XXX

THE PSYCHOLOGY OF THE INTERVIEW

THE interview is a sample of a personal relationship. Throughout this book it has been stressed that during the interview, and during all personal relationships things go on at two separate levels of the mind, the conscious and the unconscious.

What goes on at a conscious level we know by definition. That is what we mean by the conscious level. What is going on at an unconscious level, we do not know; we defend ourselves against knowing it by the process of repression. How do we know then that anything is going on at an unconscious level? What justification have we for suggesting that there is an unconscious level? The answer is that we are aware of various emotional reactions, sometimes overwhelming emotional experiences, the source or origin of which is inexplicable except on the theory of unconscious activity, except on the theory of a world of unconscious phantasies, the ideational contents of which commonly remain unconscious. Not only emotions emanate from these levels into consciousness, but also symptoms and physical reactions of every description, together with such phenomena as dreams and phantasies. Indeed, analysis has revealed that the chief motivations of our life, not excluding some of our beliefs, have their source in the unconscious mind.

But here we are chiefly concerned with the bearing of this upon the interview, and upon our relationship to persons. What brings the unconscious activities which go on at an interview so conspicuously before the mind of the analyst is not so much the interview itself, but the revelations that come about during the subsequent analysis of the patient interviewed. I mentioned in Chapter Three a patient who told me how his childhood relationship to his father was characterized by their mutual acceptance of a sort of chalk line of censorship, over which neither of them must step for fear of arousing some emotion. In the course of analysis, it transpired that this patient's principal symptom was related to this emotionally tense, personal relationship to his father, and, one might add, to a lesser extent, to his mother also. This was detectable even at his first interview with me.

He was obviously shy and embarrassed, very taut, stiff and jerky in his manner and in his speech. It was as though everything he thought or felt had to be examined by some censorship within him, some editing faculty, before it was given permission to be expressed in speech. And then, only a very stilted version of it was expressed. The chalk line precaution was clearly in operation; and this although his father had now been dead for more than twenty years.

But let us take an excerpt from his subsequent analysis as evidence of the unconscious processes at work. This man, although highly educated, was pathologically shy and introverted. That gave me the opportunity to see all the more clearly the psychopathology of such reactions, common enough in all of us. He said to me: 'It is difficult for anybody who is not like me to appreciate what an agony it has always been for me to be with people, particularly to meet people socially. Where the occasion is supposed to be one designed for pleasure, I experience it as a nightmare. All I want to do, if I cannot avoid it altogether, is to get away from it as quickly as possible.

'All through my life I have endured this nightmare. About eighteen months ago I decided I could stand it no longer. I gave up my job, as it was impossible for me to work without these agonizing personal contacts all the time, and I retreated to my dingy little basement flat. There I shut the door, as though I were shutting out the world. I heaved a sigh of relief, and tried to make my life that of a hermit. I tried to content myself with a little piano-playing, solitude, and phantasies.'

Needless to say, he had found this no solution to his problem. Depression had increased, and anxiety had not vanished. In fact, he told me that the inevitable visit from the milkman had assumed almost as gigantic proportions in its capacity for disturbing his emotions, as his contacts with the manager of his office had previously done. This showed that the real source of the trouble was internal and not external. This was the situation which had finally caused him to make an almost super-human effort, and consult a psychiatrist.

He had described his personal relationship with people as a nightmare, and, therefore, it may be worth paying a little attention to an actual nightmare which he brought me early in his treatment. He dreamt that he was in his house, associated with the flat in which he had shut himself up for so long. He saw a large group of people entering his private garden. He ran forward and ordered them out. They all left except three rather wiry and athletic men who refused to go. He entered into a struggle with these, trying to throw them out, but without success. In the course of the struggle the coat he was wearing got its lapel badly torn. His watch chain was snapped, and the watch pulled away and broken. Finally, discovering that he was physically unable to eject these men, the thought occurred to him that perhaps nothing terrible would happen if he just left them alone. He retreated into his house, and, curiously enough, found himself having a pleasurable sexual phantasy. The nightmare feeling which he had experienced in the early part of the dream had given place to one of erotic pleasure. (End of dream.)

The dream will, unfortunately, not seem so significant to the reader as it would to any analyst. Analysts are accustomed daily to dealing with dreams; they understand the cipher in which they are written, or at least they understand it with the help of the patient's association of thought to the emotional elements in the dream. Every analyst recognizes that the patient's 'house and garden' represent his own body; the numerical component 'three', ('three wiry men'), is a classical symbol representing the male genital; and the patient's 'torn garment', 'broken chain and watch', are symbolical of castration. No analyst familiar with dream symbols has any doubt about these interpretations.

The point of interest for us is that *the patient's chief symptom is that of similar feelings of anxiety, defence and attack, when he is in any social group*, particularly in any group that includes males. Of course, he does not ordinarily attack them (!), although he usually displays an unnecessary aggressiveness. There is no doubt that his ego has a struggle to behave reasonably in personal contacts with people. This is because his unconscious phantasy, like the dream, is tending to influence his behaviour with its inappropriate, irrational, but intensely compelling, emotions. In fact, this is the struggle which he had found so intolerable a strain that he had finally retreated to solitude. He felt it would be better to be alone, and shut up in his flat, than living a daily nightmare amongst people.

It may be thought that this is inadequate evidence upon which to base the psychopathology of this patient's asocial symptom and anxiety reactions in personal relationships. Perhaps it is; but I may say, space permits me to give only a small excerpt, a sample as it were of a super-abundance of material, from practically every session of this patient's analysis, all of which pointed to the same psychopathology.

The psychopathology of the nightmare may be described briefly as being caused by the dreamer's repressed feminine component seeking gratification. For this purpose it provokes the invention of a phantasy (or dream) in which some symbolic representation of the father or father's phallus (sometimes the mother's phallus), is about to overwhelm the sleeper, and thereby gratify the repressed and unconscious feminine need within him. What makes the dream a nightmare, instead of an ecstasy of gratification, is that elements in the dreamer's psyche violently oppose the wishful phantasy provoked by this feminine component. It is these other elements, nearer consciousness and more closely associated with the dreamer's ego, which feel that all will be lost (death, annihilation) unless they win in the struggle. In the nightmare they commonly feel that all *is* being lost, and, therefore, the dreamer awakes in fright, just in time to save the situation.

It transpired that this sort of thing was going on in my patient's unconscious. The social presence of males was seized upon by his unconscious phantasy to represent the attacking phallus, and this necessitated the mobilization of all his defences against the danger. What danger? The danger of his feminine component utilizing the situation for its gratification.

Now there is evidence that this phantasy of feminine-component-gratification is so strongly resisted because (as the dream and the patient's symptoms show us), it is accompanied by a phantasy of castration('torn garment', 'broken chain', 'broken watch'), and an accompanying permanent loss of masculinity, and, probably, of annihilation. The male who can enjoy the company of other males is relatively free from such alarming components in his phantasy. The father image is to him at least as security-giving, and pleasure-giving, as it is menacing.

The latter half of the dream which I have recorded is indicative of the change or modification which is coming about, as a result of the analytical movement, in the phantasy and feelings associated with personal relationships. He is even considering that it may not be necessary to fight the male, to fight father, or the symbol of father's phallus. Perhaps everything will be all right if he just leaves it alone; and lo! within his dream, everything is all right, very much all right, except for the fact that he is left somewhat 'wounded' after the unnecessary and fruitless struggle. However, from the pleasure in the latter part of the dream it would seem that his wound or injury is mended.

This particular patient had many dreams which showed most clearly the nature of *the 'nightmare' which was intruding into his social relationships* when he was awake, and causing the nightmare-feelings which resulted in his retreat.

It is only from analytical evidence, such as this, that we can begin to appreciate the fact that the emotions experienced during interviews and social relationships have their source in unconscious activity which is accompanying the conscious activity of the interview, and which may have a very illogical relationship to it. In a case such as this, where the affect (or emotion) is out of all proportion to the real and conscious relationship, we can see more clearly that it is unconscious forces, unconscious phantasies, which are responsible for these affects. Such cases are, therefore, an aid to us for demonstration purposes.

The super-abundance of such material in every patient, material of every grade of normality, and of every grade of divergence from what we regard as normal, convinces me that in every case, no matter how apparently normal, the moving factor in an interview, and in every personal relationship, is basically the unconscious factor. It is a matter of good fortune for us if our infantile and childhood experience was such that it gave us more pleasure than anxiety in our initial contacts with people. However, some anxiety is always present, and its roots are usually morbid and comparable to those that existed in the case I have been describing.

This matter will be pursued in the next chapter because it is an even deeper stage of analysis, the transference stage proper, which really brings home to us incontrovertibly that the psychology of our relationships to one another, at an interview or otherwise, lies in the unconscious processes that are at work.

CHAPTER XXXI

THE PSYCHOLOGY OF LOVE AND HATE

UNCONSCIOUS FACTORS IN PERSONAL RELATIONSHIP

THE essential ingredients of the unconscious mind are effectively and convincingly brought to consciousness only during the transference stage of analysis. It is only when a patient has experienced the transference stage, and has then had these experiences interpreted, that he recognizes clearly and incontrovertibly the truth of what has been going on unconsciously, motivating him and driving him, throughout the whole of his life. Nothing else convinces, nothing except the transference—or, more correctly, the recognition and interpretation of the transference; the analysis of it. It would seem that in the absence of transference, resistances are too strong to be broken through. On a conscious plane, we may or may not seem to believe some of the things we are told, but in any case, in so far as they are designed to throw light upon the contents of the unconscious, they can hardly be really appreciated, really understood, and really believed.

Therefore, in this chapter I am going to transcribe some transference material, the most vivid emotional material which we encounter in analysis, in the hope that this may prove more convincing to the reader than interpretations from more superficial stages of analysis.

I shall take an excerpt from a very much later stage of the analysis of the patient whose interview was described in Chapter Eighteen, an interview which I characterized as being full of understatement. It was then suggested that a great deal more was going on unconsciously than appeared on the surface. Now, in a documentary of these transference sessions, the reader will have the opportunity of seeing what it was, what was going on in this patient's unconscious during his first interview, and, indeed, throughout his life. It will be seen that it is some aspect of the emotional pattern established in infancy in relationship to the parents. Although it is quite unrealistic, and quite irrelevant to the actualities of present-day personal contacts such as interviews, it is nevertheless the source of feelings, reactions, and, to a large extent, of behaviour. These emotional patterns established in infancy are the most effective and compelling force within us, second only to our instincts. The mind cannot readily abandon them. It takes all the toil and sweat of a protracted analysis, not so much to bring them to consciousness, but to unite them so closely with the ego that some modification or change results. Here again, I am afraid that I can only give a modicum, a sample of the material at my disposal, because even the recorded portion, recorded at the time of this patient's sessions, is enough to fill several books.

At the point at which I am taking up the story, this very masculine, potentially aggressive, and heterosexual man, in the late thirties, began his session by relating the following short dream. He was not laughing so much as he was a bit startled by its evident incongruity with his nature, temperament, and character. His effective comment was, 'very odd'. The dream was simply this:
'*I was with a man whom I once knew and liked very much. This fellow was kissing me.*' The patient remarked: 'It's very odd indeed, as, like me, this man is a heterosexual fellow.' Asked what he felt in the dream, he replied, drily, 'I didn't like it very much.'

As usual, the analyst kept quiet for the patient to talk. Almost immediately he said: 'Well, I've told you how, as a child, I used to hate being kissed by my father. However, this chap was not like father at all.' After a pause, he said: 'My thought just now was that it has something to do with my analysis *here*. I think the dream must be some effort to solve the male relationship.'

One of this patient's salient difficulties in life has been that his emotional relationship to senior men has been impossibly hostile. He said: 'It is better than it used to be, but I am still a bit suspicious. I felt in the dream, "What is he wasting his time for, doing this to me, when he might be kissing a girl?" Yes, it does compare with my coming here.'

Analyst: 'Why are we wasting time with each other when you might be kissing a girl?'

Patient: 'Yes, that's it. And here we are back on the homosexual track again. Although our relationship here is only mental, the dream is describing it as an intimate physical relationship.'

Analyst: 'Perhaps all human relationships are *unconsciously* correlated with a physical emotional relationship—a sort of sexual relationship.' This particular patient's transference is characterized by resistance. He is an exceptionally 'strong-minded' person, of very independent views. The reader is not at a transference stage of analysis, but, nevertheless, I would like him, like the patient, to take note of what I said to this patient. The freedom of the analyst's remarks, so different from that in interviews and in early sessions, should be explained. It is due to two things: one, that this ground has been covered before *by the patient*, and two, transference calls for free interpretation by the analyst. This patient, though commonly distinguished by a tendency to disagreement with everything I say, in this instant simply said, 'Yes.'

That encouraged me to continue: 'From the fact that all human relationships are unconsciously correlated with a physical relationship can be better understood the affects (emotions) that accompany them.'

Patient: 'Yes, I was resistant to it. Not only was I resistant to my father's kisses—oh, horrible things!—but to anything and everything associated with him. If he gave me a ball to play with, I was resistant. I did not want the money he left me. I could not enjoy it. They were all parts of him, and I wanted to reject the lot —lock, stock and barrel. That is why I wanted to get away from home—as far as possible; like I want to get away from you.'

Analyst: 'Every dealing with your father was unconsciously identified with an unwelcome sexual intimacy with him?'

Patient: 'Yes, that's right; every damned thing about him. If I accepted anything from him, it gave me a feeling of inferiority.'

Analyst: 'His intimacy was unwelcome because it was related to castration feelings.'

'Yes, I see that. But then, why the hell do I have a dream of him, or rather of you, disguised in the form of a friend, kissing me?'

Analyst: 'Does the dream suggest you *could* have an intimacy with father provided you could feel secure against castration?'

'Yes, that's right. I have been thinking that it might be all right for me to have a job, provided I could be my own boss.'

The patient began his next session with his familiar rantings and ravings against 'being dragged back' to 'this blessed office' every day. He shouted: 'I am fed up with it. I want to be free.' My interpretation was—'Your phantasy is that you are being asked to submit to father, to father's being intimate with you, and evidently at the same time castrating you. One part of your mind is producing the phantasy, and the other part is fighting it.'

Patient: 'One part of my mind is ignoring it, and the other part is conscious of it all the time.'

Analyst, interpreting the unconscious phantasy: 'Father is doing something good to you, gratification, and you are enjoying it, and yielding to the temptation of it, acquiescing. Suddenly you realize that the result of this gratification is that you will be castrated, emasculated, or annihilated, and so you turn from acquiescing, and start resisting—as it were, fighting for your life, fighting against the temptation of yielding to father.'

The patient only remarked: 'I suppose there are other families about like ours, who were so damnably possessive that you had practically to murder them to get away from them.'

In the meantime I was thinking that in his dream the *form* of the intimacy had been oral, and perhaps inadequate reference had been made to this, so I added: 'Possessiveness may be at an earlier emotional level than the genital, and in your dream, the intimacy is a kissing one. Therefore, we could say that the relationship with father is at an oral level, possibly connected with incorporation and destruction.'

However, what a patient has to say is always more interesting than anything the analyst can say. This patient continued, just speaking his own thoughts, as he usually did. He said: 'Everything is all right. Father is kissing me. *Then* I find that the price I have to pay for the kissing is following-in-his-footsteps, being a beastly clergyman like him, doing the same work as he does, having my life commandeered by him.' And then suddenly this patient shouted, '*Having no life of my own.*'

This was interpreted as annihilation, and counter-annihilation expressed as shouting (c.f. a baby's screaming). He said: 'For *my* personality, this possession, this incorporation, was death. It was not ordinary family ties they wanted. It was all-encompassing. England is not far enough away from Belfast. I shall never be well until I am thousands of miles away. This kissing may have been something good, but the sequel would be to obey the law of the patriarch, to be possessed, swallowed by father, and that would be death, annihilation.

'It was either that reaction to the family, accepting annihilation, or the reaction which I have shown. I have something in me that when it is touched off—phew! up it goes. I blow the whole thing up. That is why I have fought all the father-figures in my life. The amazing thing is that I have gone on coming to you. I think I come really to fight you. I have to fight to prevent myself from being swallowed up. My tragedy is that as an infant something good was offered me (c.f. the kissing). Then I looked round, and found that for that good, I had to sign myself away. I can see that I have been acting out this sort of thing all my life, and am still doing so. It needs something more than analysis to stop it. How is it ever going to change?'

I here departed from the usual technique of interpretation in order to be a little didactic, and therefore replied as follows: 'With *sufficient* insight the ego cannot help taking over more and more of it, instead of being taken over by it. It is not a question of *effortful* interference by the ego. The emotions go on, but the ego increasingly *looks* on, and decreasingly enters into it. The ego no longer *has* to enter the emotional vortex. We all have emotional reactive patterns which we accept as part of ourselves, unfortunate parts perhaps, but the fruit of analysis is that we are not deluded or taken in by them, nor necessarily unduly disturbed by the fact that they exist.'

Patient, shouting: 'I have got *feelings*. They are feelings of towards, and feelings of resistance. What can be done about that?' After a pause, he continued, more quietly, 'I see it all, and I see that the ego has taken over to a remarkable extent, considering the condition I was in; but I have had a hell of a life, owing to this conflict in me, created by my parents. (I know you won't have that.) It has prevented my doing the things I would otherwise have liked to do. I can't help being angry about it.'

It will be seen that this patient is the victim of a phantasy, or emotional pattern, developed in infancy. It would seem that at first there were elements of the 'good' parent (probably mother) to whom he was instinctually attracted (hence the dream of the kiss), and, perhaps subsequently, a very powerful phantasy of the 'bad' parent (largely father) who would swallow, destroy or annihilate him. The conflict at this very deep level, which might be regarded as a conflict between love and hate at an *instinctual* level, becomes clearer, as a conflict at a *structural* level, between id—largely identified with himself (ego)—and super-ego. The latter is largely projected on to the father-image.

Then there emerges what would appear to be the main conflict of his life: the phantasy of a most bitter struggle, as it were to the death, between himself (largely his id) and the father-image.

His dream of the kiss is clearly an attempt to reconcile these two, to unite 'Self' and 'Father', and dissolve their antagonism. In so far as I am the man kissing him, he is using me, through the transference, to dramatize this much-wished-for reconciliation. In so far as the conflict is basically intrapsychic the dream can be regarded as his super-ego and id kissing each other, and so ending their long, exhausting enmity. The conflict ends, and they live happily ever after.

It here occurs to me to say that the phenomenon of *falling-in-love*, about which too little has been written by psycho-analysts and too much left to novelists, is, in my opinion, like this kissing, largely, perhaps principally, an attempt to unite the conflicting Super-ego and Id, and so dissolve the painful, exile-maintaining conflict. It will be conceded that there is usually little tendency for a person to fall in love with someone essentially symbolizing the id. Though he may be sexually attracted, the man does not tend to *fall in love* principally with 'dirty' 'sluts' and prostitutes, and the woman with men of a 'lower' (i.e. more 'id') class. The tendency is to conceive of the loved one as 'pure', 'clean', 'superior' or 'perfect' in some way or another. In fact we are in love with them and want them largely because they are so 'excellent' or wonderful; that is to say because they are so super-egoish; and we hope that, nevertheless, they may allow our humble id to unite with them. The 'oceanic feeling' of psychosexual consummation that some psycho-analysts talk about is unscientifically vague, and I think would be more precisely and more accurately understood by this concept of a symbolic union of id and super-ego, a union in which the agony of 'war', anxiety, hate and exile comes to an end, the antagonism of id and super-ego ceases, 'child' and 'parent' are reconciled and peace reigns for evermore within the mind and without. They are married 'and live happily ever after.'

I have a hunch that *full* psychosexual orgasm ('the Cinderella of the sciences'), for which we have known men and women travel from one end of the Earth to the other (as though there were no possible mate nearer!), and sacrifice their all, even their lives, is nothing more or less than the complete consummation of this all-important reconciliation.

All this is by no means irrelevant to the psychology of the interview. Similar if not identical phantasies are being dramatized in an attenuated form, however unconsciously, during the interview. Most commonly, the Interviewer becomes, by projection, the super-ego, and the Interviewed identifies himself with the id. It is relevant because the Interviewer should have enough insight to safeguard him from compulsively subscribing to this projection; and the Interviewed should (ideally) be sufficiently free from conflict between his id and super-ego to be free from 'nerves', anxiety and aggression, and free also from dependence and surrender-tendencies. In other words he should be sufficiently comfortable to deal appropriately with the reality situation. This means he should be free from the compulsion to use the persons and 'props' of the interview-situation as vehicles for the acting out of his unresolved conflicts. He never is!

CHAPTER XXXII

TRANSFERENCE

A PECULIARITY of the transference stage of analysis, or rather of a late stage of the transference, is that emotions and early patterns of emotion are not only transferred on to the person of the analyst, but are felt with extraordinary vividness, as though they really belonged there. The most inappropriate feelings for and about the analyst are felt and believed to have at last found their appropriate focus! Moreover the patient often, though by no means always, expresses them with a freedom which would have been impossible at an earlier stage. Aggression and hate, no less than dependence and love, are freely unloaded.

The patient, whose Oedipus Complex (in the form of transference) was being discussed in the last chapter, aptly stigmatized the free and voluble outpouring of his aggression as 'blowing-off'. He shouted it out at the top of his voice: *'I am sick of coming here, and not getting any satisfaction. I don't want to be tamed, to be made dead like all the other castrated or half-dead people in the world. It is death or partial death, that I am fighting. I'm not dead; not yet. I am not tamed. I shall blow off as much as I like. Blowing off is ME.'*

Having discharged these sentiments with a violence and volume of sound that almost made the windows vibrate, he was quiet for a few moments. Then he said softly: 'There is a *hard knot* in me that produces these emotions. While the knot is there, I have no appetite. I would say that for two years I have been "sicking something up".'

After a silence, I said to him: 'By "hard knot" do you mean something tied-up?'

He said: 'Yes, it's like a tied-up spring in me.'

Analyst: 'Is that what, in the jargon, we would call "conflict"?'

Patient: 'Yes, that's right.'

Analyst: 'What are the two opposing elements in this conflict or "hard knot"?'

Patient: 'One says, "stop this blowing-off, and settle down, and be like other people", and the other says, "not on your life, that would be death". The other wants to have it. It just gets angry and blows off all the louder.'

Analyst: 'When you blow off you are discharging one half of the "knot". The other side of this "knot" is?'

Patient: 'It's the part that says I should not. The knot is looser, but it is still there. Two years ago I felt it more.

'You might say it is trying to get out while something else is stopping it. I am not feeling it so much now. It is as though there were a wall, and I had partly got through it, but not completely.

'My wife is coming back from a holiday with her mother, but I don't want her to come back yet. There is something more important, more urgent to be done at the moment; and I can only deal with one thing at a time. I am still a bit restless.'

Analyst: 'There was a time when you restlessly travelled about all over the world? What were you trying to do then?'

Patient: 'Oh, I suppose I was trying to get away from this blessed knot, like a man trying to get away from his shadow. No, I didn't enjoy anything. As you say, I travelled about, I ran about, but I had a knot inside me all the time. I was struggling to ignore it. I was a sick man pretending to be well, going through the motions of living.'

He then proceeded to sum up: 'One thing in me is saying, "you can't go on doing this irrational blowing-off, you have *got* to stop it", and something else says, "I damn well *will*!" ' He added, 'And I think it is unravelling it somehow. I think it is, I don't know how. I feel it is going to cease one day, and then I shall feel grand. I do, in fact, feel a good deal better.'

Incidentally, I may say that this remark of his is a little heartening for his analyst, for he is the last man generally to admit such a thing; his emotional gratification is usually obtained by shouting the opposite.

He continued: 'I now feel we are dealing with the residue. It has been loosened a lot, but something is still kicking. There is an internal frustration which I felt very keenly two years ago, and all my life before that. I do not feel it so strongly now—just the remnants. How much more of this can we get rid of? My wife is irrelevant to the whole situation. Any so-called adjustments, such as I was trying restlessly before I came to analysis, are all irrele-

vant. You tell your patients from me that everything they do outside their analytical sessions, work or anything else, is irrelevant.
At the most, or the worst, it means that *that* part of them which
finds adjustment outside will never be analysed. Therefore, they
are only cheating analysis by trying to find adjustment outside.
Every extra-analytical adjustment is irrelevant.'

In other words, he is now, at the end of his session, voicing a
conviction the very opposite from that with which he started it. He
started by saying 'I am sick of coming here, and not getting anywhere.' He finishes, more or less as usual, by saying: 'Anything
other than coming here to these sessions is irrelevant.'

He arrived at his next session, calm, cool, and collected, and
announced that his wife had returned, and he had had sexual intercourse with her. Perhaps his calmness and sanity rather under-
lined his parting statement of the day before (that she and everything outside analysis were 'irrelevant'), in the sense that he did
not have the usual emotional pressure, or dynamic force, behind
the analytical expression of his thoughts and feelings.

Presently, however, he lapsed into criticisms of his wife. This
defensive projection was getting us nowhere, and so I interjected:
'It is not that your wife, or indeed anything outside yourself,
creates your emotional situation. On the other hand, it has become
clear to us in the course of these two years that your wife is the
environment or "object" in which and upon which you *act out* the
various facets of your internal conflicts.'

The patient said: 'Yes, that's right. I suppose in a way I have
recognized it, and that is why I have not tried to choose another. I
just make her into an alternating gratification and castration,
according to which side of my conflict is uppermost. It is just my
way of going on living. The only way I know. Perhaps her going
away for a bit allowed the conflict to rest a little. Generally I am
just going on with it, or them (or inhibiting them), in my relationship to any person I may be with. Look how I do it with
you!'

The patient and I were both able to see pretty clearly that 'going on living' meant acting out our complexes, internal emotional
conflicts and pressures, in relationship to persons and things
around us. I would like the reader to take note of this, as this is
one of the essential lessons which this book has to teach us. Uncon-

sciously we are doing this acting out in all our personal relationships, even at the interview. However, it may have been owing to his wife's return that very little of special emotional interest transpired during that particular session.

At his next session things were warming up again slightly. He complained that he found he could not do anything without conflict. He said: 'That is why it is no good my preparing to go away on a holiday. Something is going on inside me all the time. It is the *knot* inside me all the time. I think my id is forever encountering my super-ego. I don't know what other people get, whether they too have a conflict like mine. Something wants to come out. Something wants to take something over, and I won't let it. I am sitting on it. I think it is because I know from experience that whatever I take over, whatever hobby or pleasure, even fishing, my blessed super-ego will take it out of my hands, so that, for instance, I would have to go on fishing day and night trying to catch more than any other person had ever done, until, finally, I threw the whole blessed thing, rod and all, into the river, and had done with it! It has been the same with everything I have taken up. It becomes a sort of super-ego task, and then I lose the taste for it. I am sure that it all goes back to my bloody parents, but I don't want to examine that. I don't want to be bothered with any bloody task. I just want to *blow off*—and *murder* the lot.'

It is noteworthy that in infancy this patient suffered from tantrums, and I am convinced that these tantrums were, even at the tender age of three, like his present-day 'blowings-off', the symbolical 'murder' of his parents. It has rightly been said that every appreciable neurosis or psychosis has a counterpart in infancy.

However much disparaged by patients and others, dreams have been called by Freud the 'royal road to the unconscious.' Having this patient's last dream in mind, I said to him: 'The energy that wants to get out is an aggressive reaction against being annihilated, an aggressive reaction against your father's "castrating", emasculating, or annihilating intimacy.'

He said: 'Yes, it's aggressive energy, always wanting to come out, and something's sitting on top of it. For instance, with my wife, something says "be nice", and something else is saying, "be damned to it". I hate you too, because you are saying as it were, that I can't let out my aggression. If I can't let out my aggression, if I hold it in, I get a knot in my stomach, and that knot is going to lead to duodenal ulcer. I can feel it. So you are condemning me to duodenal ulcer, to death. That is why I am fighting you and all the "fathers". I'm fighting for my life.' (This attitude may not be so irrational as it sounds.)

At his next session, he started by complaining of his so-called marital duties to his wife. He said: 'I had a bad night, after intercourse. Before it, I thought to myself, "*I* shan't get any pleasure out of this." That is the curse of marriage. You take on a thing, and then it becomes a sort of castrating duty. As I told you before, if I took up even fishing it would become that in my case. Anyhow, I think it is so with most people. There must be an awful lot of this *duty* intercourse going on. It has a bad effect. After it, I awoke at four-thirty a.m. with this pain. I got up, and made myself a cup of tea. That helped a bit.'

I may mention here that this sort of thing had happened before, and had been related to hunger-screamings in his babyhood. These were eventually relieved by the overdue feed, now symbolized by the cup of tea.

He said: 'After the tea I went to sleep again, and I had a curious dream, or rather two dreams in succession.'

As the unconscious phantasy is the source of our emotions, our symptoms, and our symptomatic behaviour, and as the dream is its codified transcription in consciousness, it is not incorrect to say that we are unwittingly *experiencing and living our 'dreams'*, without knowing their conceptual content. Knowledge of this content, when we can acquire it, often provides a surprising and unsuspected explanation of everything which previously seemed inexplicable. The dreams of this patient, as of every patient and of every person, are sufficiently illuminating to deserve a terminal chapter to themselves.

CHAPTER XXXIII

WE ARE UNWITTINGLY LIVING
OUR DREAMS

THE dreams, referred to in the last chapter, and their analysis are worth our attention as they confirm my theory that something goes on in the unconscious in every personal relationship, including the interview, something unsuspected by consciousness, something the affects or emotions of which are the essential psychological ingredient of the personal relationship, and the effective force influencing our reactions, our conduct, and even our thoughts.

The first of the two dreams, dreamt consecutively on that night, was related by the patient as follows: 'There was a bronze horse, and a black one. The black one jumped on top of the other one, and I thought, "These horses are going to get out of control." The black one was biting the neck of the other. I thought, "They are going to knock everything over—*Look Out!*" In other words, I got that sudden acute anxiety feeling, the "look-out" feeling which I get in some of my dreams, but in this case I did not wake up with it. Instead, the horse got off the other one, and everything was all right.

'Immediately I went on to dream quite a different dream: I am with an older man, a man whom I knew in my University days and liked very much. I said something, and he contradicted me. Then I am with you and another fellow. I think we are having some sort of argument. You said: "You won't always be friends, you know."' The patient added: 'I think it is to do with some sort of strain between the two of us.'

The point of interest about this dream material is the fact that these two dreams were on the same night, in sequence. Dreams of the same night are always about the same latent dream-thought, either a repetition, or a continuation or a sequel, one of the other. The censorship or defence-resistance activity is very conspicuous in the fact that the sexual-intercourse-element, in the first dream, has been, as it were, deliberately separated from the relationship-to-the-analyst-element, as depicted in the second dream, or, more truthfully, the second part of the same dream. We shall see the significance of this presently.

In association to the dream, the patient said: 'In the actual sexual intercourse which I had before the dream, I first satisfied my wife (duty), and then I turned her over, and had intercourse with her from behind to satisfy myself, or *to try* to satisfy myself. Perhaps I was a bit rough and sadistic. Anyhow, after it she burst into tears.

'I don't know what woke me up at four-thirty in the morning, whether it was that I had not been psychologically satisfied with her, or whether it was my damned super-ego, giving me a bad time for my bad behaviour. I was restless. I felt awful; like I'd felt in the horses-nightmare. Anyhow, the horses in the dream obviously refer to what had just taken place, *that bit of intercourse*. I must have got worried, although I would not have remembered it but for the dream "look-out", just before the end.' Then he said a surprising and significant thing: 'I think the disturbance, which woke me up, is due to some sort of thing *that goes on in this analysis*, the damned therapeutic, clinical approach (!), as a result of which I get *no satisfaction*.'

With this, the patient started tossing himself about, showing extreme restlessness, suggestive of the sort of emotion that had given rise to the nightmare and that had awakened him at four-thirty in the morning. I said: 'You appear to be showing some conflict *now*, at this moment.'

He 'got it' all right, and replied immediately: 'I agree with you. I wonder how much it is *you*. It is like bringing you things, bringing things to you and father. My *id* says, "You are just doing this sex for father"; and then I don't want to do it at all. What I am really wanting to do is to tell father, and you, to go to hell.'

He went on, very rightly, to say what I had been thinking but deliberately refraining from saying, in the hope that he would say it first: 'If we analysed the reactions between *you and me*, and left all these other people out of it, we would get on a damned sight better and faster. The trouble is that I have lost the feeling for intercourse, *because* all the time I am being used sexually by father, and castrated. Even if I try to have some intercourse on my own account, it is irrelevant, it is meaningless. What really fills the whole field is this relationship between you and me. The other is all off-the-mark. That is why, the more I go in for anything like this, such as intercourse with my wife, all I get is this feeling of tension. When my wife was away, I could get down to the business of "knocking-your-block-off". Now she has come back, we are missing the point.'

Analyst: 'The point is "me"?'

Patient: 'All my reactions are reactions to you. There must be either active attack or passive resistance, but always to *you*. I am resistant to you when I am telling you dreams, because I am not getting my gratification by telling you dreams, I am submitting to you, to your "technique". There is only a free flow when I am blowing-off, dealing with you, fighting you, instead of submitting to your forcing your intimacies upon me. Of course, what happened last night was only a waste of time, like all the other things outside analysis. It was only an attempt at escape, a fruitless attempt. I wish I could get my wife out of the way, and get down to dealing with my father. I feel I have been assaulted sexually, and so I feel I have to go off and do some sex myself—perhaps to get even, to try and reassure myself or mend myself. It is no good. It is not an enjoyment; it is a strain. That's the strain I felt when I awoke in the night. Every time I come back here to you, my feelings interpret it as submitting to your doing something to me.'

Analyst: '*Essentially* you are in some struggle with *me*?'

'Yes, and in the midst of that struggle, I go off, and have intercourse with my wife; and at four-thirty in the morning I wake up, and feel, "What have I done"? Somehow it would seem as though by my action I had given you some advantage in the struggle. I should not have wasted my energies. They should all have been mobilized for the struggle with you. It is as though a country that was at war, went off and wasted its energy in an attempt to get some ridiculous pleasure. It's crazy. I woke up in the morning feeling as though I had done something crazy. I felt I had let myself down, and as a result you might get the better of me. On the other hand, when I am blowing-off here, I get the opposite of that feeling. Often in the past I felt, "I will keep away from sex, so that I can beat the hell out of this chap (you)."

'My relationship to you is the essence of the whole conflict. On the other hand, it seems that my super-ego is saying to me, "You go along and submit to being assaulted sexually by father", and I come along! but instead of submitting, I keep objecting; for, against all this, there is my *id* which has mobilized all this energy to fight you and beat you, and then that would be the end. The "knot" in my stomach is a struggle with father. It has no relevance to my having intercourse with my wife. Any activity outside my relationship to you, such as intercourse with my wife, is tantamount to admitting defeat. It is like saying, "I can't get past father, so I will dodge him"; and something else in me says, until I can come here without any diversion of my interest and energy, I have not scotched father. Something says, "You have either got to murder father, or leave him". To leave father would be to run out. That is what I tried to do all my life before I came to analysis; running out of the battle is no good, so I come back here for more. To win or to die fighting; but never to submit. Yet I suppose I must have submitted in some way, or I would not be better. And I would hardly have dreamt that dream of the kiss.'

Briefly these dreams reveal the unconscious phantasy of an intimate sexual relationship to the analyst, he having displaced the parent and become the parent image. This sexual relationship is full of frustration, fear, aggression and reactive hate. Nevertheless, it is the one really strong emotional pattern and it compulsively repeats and expresses itself in all his personal relationships as is vividly shown in his relationship to his analyst. The value of this material, from an analytical point of view, is not so much the interpretation of it, the tying of it all together in a logical bundle, but the mere fact that it is coming out, that the patient is expressing it, together with its related emotions. In other words, it is reaching his conscious level, albeit in all sorts of disguised forms. In his second part of the dream, for example, he introduced many displacements. Although I, his analyst, do appear in the end, even I myself am clearly a displacement of the father, and also to some extent of the mother, of his early life.

In short, he is giving expression, bringing to consciousness, the various facets of his Oedipus complex, of the emotional pattern which was formed in infancy in his relationship to his mother and father, an emotional pattern which was full of hate, projected hate, and reactive hate and aggression. These reactions proved too strong to leave him in peace to react rationally or even normally to situations throughout his life. They are particularly strongly stimulated by personal relationships. That is why he is largely a recluse in spite of, or perhaps because of, his very strong and sensitive emotional 'appreciation' of every personal relationship.

He once said to me that he found contact with people *too* stimulating. He could only safeguard himself against this too great stimulation by withdrawing from contact. That is largely because what this contact stimulates is an unconscious pattern, an Oedipus pattern, which it is impracticable to express. His ego, his reason, knows that he cannot go to social Clubs and spend his time 'knocking the blocks off' all the people—and they would be the majority —who stimulate him adversely at the moment.

He can be, and often is, positively stimulated also, but there is always the danger that some remark, some indiscretion, some tactlessness, on the other person's part will provoke a storm of aggression. If he succeeds in suppressing the aggressive impulses, he himself will be occupied with nothing but their suppression, and will have no emotional interest or energy left over for the expected ordinary personal relationships. He will feel the knot in his stomach more acutely, and will come away from the situation with more intolerable tension, and he will be feeling ill with it. But, worse than this, from an external point of view, is the fact that he may not be able completely to control the aggressive urges, as their strength and violence is so phenomenal. It only requires a modicum of such impulses to break through, and every person in his vicinity will recognize, at least subconsciously, that he is holding in him the inadmissible, the prohibited world of hate and destruction. It will electrify the atmosphere—because everyone else is holding it in also—desperately repressing it.

He is a frank, open man and does not stoop to the customary subtle methods of discharge, or gratification, of aggressive impulses by the usual conventional subterfuges. He would be more likely to shout at his adversary, though equally ready to make friends afterwards. It does not work in society. That is what he has found.

In the course of his analysis he found also that the whole thing emanates from infantile stresses, and from what he, rightly or wrongly, felt as his parents' responsibility for them. Those were his earliest, his initial personal contacts, and these later ones, like

that with his analyst, are only *stimulations of the original pattern.*
There is one other point I wish to make in this chapter. Transference is always ambivalent, a mixture of love and hate, of
libido and aggression, of life instincts and death instincts. Interpretations, other than interpretations of resistances, are usually pretty
futile until the transference stage of analysis has arrived. Analysis
proper begins with the transference; analysis is interpretation and
analysis of the transference. Until the transference has been established, the analyst is pretty helpless as a therapeutic power. If he
does not know that fact, he will remain a 'surface' analyst. But, even
with this effective power, namely the transference, one finds that
the mind is most reluctant to give up the expression, the dramatizing and acting-out, of its emotional patterns. *In this respect, they
are, in my opinion, comparable to instincts, although of later development. In acting them out, as in achieving the aim of an instinct, the
individual is experiencing gratification, perhaps the only sort of gratification which he can experience.*

*My patient has equated it with life, and he has equated the demand
for its alteration or modification with death or partial death. The
organism is most reluctant to give up the gratification of its instincts,
and the individual is most reluctant to give up the acting out of his
(infantile) emotional pattern, in favour of ego development.* Like the
infant, he will only do this, or even attempt to do it, out of fear,
or in exchange for, as it were, the 'love' of the parent or parent
figure.

It is through the first personal relationships, through introjecting the good parent figures, that the growing individual can
tolerate some sacrifice of instinct gratification. It is only *through
the transference,* and successful analysis of the transference, *that the
patient can forego the acting out of his Oedipus complex, in favour of
ego development.* Even so, such a change, however small, is resisted
all along, as though it were a 'castrating' or life-depriving process.
Freud has related ego-development to a 'desexualization'. This
can obviously be equated with the concept of a 'castration' of
pleasure.

However, with the introduction of the Oedipus patterns, through
transference interpretation and analysis, into consciousness so that
they come under the auspices of the patient's ego, certain modifications automatically take place, and the ego effects a better

adaptation between their demands and those of environmental reality.

This is the nature of the unconscious forces, of which the individual has no cognizance, which are effectively intruding into all his personal relationships, including that of the first interview. How far they normally are from conscious appreciation, can perhaps be better realized by a study of the documentary which I have transcribed in these chapters.

How fully the analyst, or for that matter any interviewer, must be aware of them and of their nature in his own personal psyche before he can be relied upon to discount them subjectively, and to appreciate them objectively (i.e. in the interviewed), I must leave to the reader to conjecture.

CHAPTER XXXIV

POSTCRIPT

THERE are so many relevant matters left out of this book that I shall not attempt to outline them. It was my intention to compile only an introduction, not a compendium. The subject of human relationships appears to be limitless and to extend into every nook and cranny of all that is human, not only into psychology, but, all even more obviously, into sociology and anthropology; they are intimately concerned with the relationship of one person to another.

In this book I aspired merely to indicate that such relationships have little of reality and of rationality in them compared with the enormous quantity of dynamic emotional motivation, instinctual and acquired, particularly acquired in our first relationships to the first people who intruded into the earliest years, months, weeks and hours of our dawning life. For our first individual reactions, even to inanimate matter and part-objects, had much to do with the establishing of reactive patterns which laid the foundation of subsequent, more elaborate reactions to whole-objects, persons and personalities. Analysis consists largely in bringing to light the source of our reactions—all of them; though it is the inappropriate ones that may strike us more forcefully.

I had a patient, a young actor, who consulted me principally on account of the disadvantageous inappropriateness of his reactions at first interviews and in other personal relationships. He said: 'When I have to interview a prospective employer, such as a producer, particularly if he is an important man from my point of view, particularly if I am very keen to get the vacancy he may have to offer, I behave in the most disastrously inappropriate manner. Instead of showing myself off as the confident and capable actor I know I am, I behave like a small boy before the most august parent. In fact, it *is* just as I used to behave *as* a small boy in front of my parents, of whom I was terrified. I give him, my interviewer, the floor, as it were, instead of taking it myself. I suppose underneath, I really want to take the *door*, not the floor,

H

and I succeed in being given it, or shown it, in the end! I become very quiet, I wait for him to speak and I say just 'Yes' and 'No.' The result is that although *I* know I could fill the vacancy perfectly, I don't get the job. Who wants a self-obliterating actor?

'In childhood I was taught that small boys should be seen and not heard, and I learnt that role so well that it requires more effort than I am capable of to counter the teaching when I find myself confronted by a producer as important to me now as my parents were then. Of course, if the man is small-fry and I don't particularly want the lousy job he has to offer, *then* I am splendid! I can jump on chairs and tables and spout away about everything . . . and I get the lousy job! In truth this is the reason why I always get the small jobs that I don't want, and miss the big opportunities.' How many of us suffer from similar ineptitudes!

I am tempted to go a stage further with this man's case-material just to convince the reader that he is, like all of us, reacting to (inherited and acquired) emotional patterns in his personal relationships, at the expense of appropriate reality-reactions. For instance, he complains bitterly that in his relationships to the opposite sex he is compulsively driven by a complex which, despite his insight, he cannot resist or counter. To begin with he cannot successfully approach, or take the initiative with, a woman just because she attracts him and he likes her. It is almost as though something in his mind said: 'What has *that* got to do with anything?' We common people do not approach princesses or queens because they are attractive. It is out of the question; indeed the question does not arise.

On the other hand if a woman, particularly an older woman, is attracted *to* him, or takes the initiative in approaching him, he is almost compulsively at her service. It is as though his queen had given him a command! Nevertheless, putting himself at her disposal, as it were, is not necessarily an unmitigated pleasure for him. On the contrary, very often it is the opposite. It is fear, not pleasure, that drives him to do her bidding, that puts him in the service of her slightest and greatest behest. It is hers to command; he would not dare to disobey, and one of his 'duties' is to see that he plays with apparent verve and delight the part she allots him. Mere willingness would not be enough if it is her pleasure that he should enjoy pleasing her.

This process can go to any length. If she wants him to make love to her he must do it with the appropriate semblance of enthusiasm and passion. Unfortunately, even his love-life thereby becomes for him more a duty and a task than a happiness or a joy. He says: 'Always I have to put "myself", my own feelings, entirely out of the picture in favour of the very doubtful compensation of knowing that I am doing what the woman desires. I don't want to be like this. It is as though complying with her wishes outweighed every other consideration. What *I* want or feel matters nothing in comparison to what she wants. Is it because I am afraid to be otherwise? Am I afraid to say "no" to a woman, or even to let her suspect any unwillingness in me?' It is! Fear is a compelling emotion that takes precedence over all others.

It was not long before this patient (as I had anticipated) was telling me how as a small boy he was terrified of his hysterical mother. He said: 'My one anxiety was to fall in with everything she wanted immediately. I was terrified that at any moment there might be an emotional storm, that she might fly into a temper; and then goodness knows what would happen. It seems to me now that *I* had to be the adult, keeping her sweet, as it were, because *she* was the hysterical child.'

He is still the adult-child or child-adult behaving 'reasonably' or 'as requested' towards the otherwise-terrifying mother-figures of his present-day life. He has not even learnt how to escape them, or how to escape or to counter the compelling force of those early emotional patterns, laid down by fear, during his infancy and childhood. His personal relationships, like his interviews, have been conditioned in his early relationships to his, long-since deceased, mother. The truth is that all of *ours* (interviews and personal relationships) have been similarly conditioned, and similarly are relatively little affected by the requirements of reason and reality. Indeed, in his case, his reactions are little affected by his own pleasure-requirements either. Even his desires have been put away, brushed aside, by the over-riding need to keep fear out.

Fortunately, we are not all in such bad fettle, but the principle remains true for us all, namely, that inherited and acquired patterns of reaction determine our personal relationships at interviews, and in all circumstances, despite our relatively impotent and effortful attempts to counter them in favour of reason.

The presence of another person is usually too stimulating a situation, too stimulating to the old-established reactive patterns, for the newly-acquired, embryonic, faculty of reason to dominate, or indeed to play anything but a very minor role. Conditioned reactive patterns, based upon instincts, if not conditioned reflexes, predominate in our relationships to one another, whether or not they beguile our ego or reason into believing that they are appropriate.

From time immemorial the presence of another member of our own species was a specific stimulus to our most important mental reactions. It commonly spelt fight, flight, 'herd-instinct', companionship, security or sexuality. Reason is usually a very weak counter to such phylogenetically entrenched reactions, so weak indeed that it is most usually their servant rather than their master. We actually believe that our instinctual reactions are rational and appropriate, when often the most that can be said for them is that they discharge our tensions and produce feelings of gratification, thereby making us, and sometimes others, willing victims of their seduction.

It is on this account that the extrovert seeks the company of others; and it is on account of his difficulty in attaining gratifications of this sort, and on account of suffering the opposite of gratification, such as the stimulation of tension and anxiety without relief, that the introvert shuns his fellow beings. His alternative is to endure the discomfort of their presence. There can of course be an infinite variety of reactions between these two extremes as well as specific reactions according to the particular person or persons responsible for the stimulus. In all of them reason plays a very small part indeed. It is often either obliterated or tagged-on, like 'an advocate for the defence', to justify or rationalize our predetermined tension-reducing reactions.

Indeed, many chapters might be written to show that the highly prized, and rightly highly prized, and rare, quality of reason has in each of us been largely vitiated by the seducing and threatening effects of our unconscious, compelling emotional patterns. I have documented clinical material all through this book to demonstrate how the unconscious mind, with its reservoir of instincts and emotional reactive patterns, determines our reactions to one another, our behaviour, and even our thoughts, beliefs and reasonings.

The capacity to reason objectively is a faculty that emerges most painfully and slowly in the course of evolution, from the established reactive patterns laid down through hundreds of millions of years of physical, chemical, physiological and instinctual reactions to the forces, personal and otherwise, that impinge upon us from within and from without. A capacity for true, objective reasoning is merely the spearhead of our most recent adaptations to environment. In personal relationships, the old forces, hundreds of millions of years strong, are usually too much for it, if there is any portion of it untainted by their influence.

GLOSSARY

Abreaction—The re-experiencing of repressed emotional tension.

Aetiology—The science of causation.

Affect—The energy of an emotion. It may be aroused by a variety of stimuli and is capable of displacement on to concepts with which it was not originally associated.

Allergies—Illnesses due to a hypersensitiveness of body cells to one or more specific proteins.

Alloerotic—The adjective of allo-erotism; erotism directed to another person.

Ambivalence—The simultaneous existence of opposing affects, such as love and hate, directed towards the same person or object. One or both of the affects may be unconscious.

Amnesia—A memory blank.

Analysand—One who is being treated by analysis.

Antibiotics—The name given to a new series of therapautic agents, prepared from cultures of living organisms, which are detrimental to the life of certain other organisms. The principal antibiotics are penicillin, chloromycetin, aureomycin, etc.

Auto-Erotism—Self-generated erotic stimulation without resort to another person.

Biosphere—The sphere of living organisms, both plants and animals. Prof. Sir J. Arthur Thompson recognises three great 'Orders of Facts': The Cosmosphere of non-living forces and things, the Biosphere of living organisms and the Sociosphere of human societary forces acting as units.

Castration—Removal of the organs of generation.

Cannabalism—The eating of one's kind. There is psycho-analytical evidence that onto-genetically as well as phylogenetically the individual passes through a stage, associated with the development of teeth, at which he 'deals with' persons and the affects they arouse in him by the phantasy of devouring them.

Clinical—Originally of or pertaining to the sick-bed and hence to do with observation of the actual patient, as distinct from theoretical constructions.

Complex—A group of affectively charged ideas which, through conflict, have become repressed into the unconscious.

Conflict—'War' between opposing elements in the mind.

Cyclothymia—A condition characterised by recurring phases of elation and depression, its extreme form being manic-depressive psychosis.

Death Instinct—According to Freud, a deeply rooted instinctual impulse that serves to take the organism back as far as possible to its original inorganic state. It is supposed to be closely associated with destructive, aggressive and repetitive tendencies in the psyche, and to contrast with the 'life' or libidinal instinct.

Defence Resistance—All contrivances, conscious and unconscious, employed by a person to avoid insight into his motivations, or specifically by an analysand to retard the progress of his analysis.

Displacement—The transfer of an affect from the idea to which it was originally attached to an associated idea. It is one of the most important unconscious mechanisms in the production of phobias and other symptoms.

Ego—That part of the id which has become modified by the impingement of external stimuli in such a way that it has become adapted to reality, reality testing and activity, and is credited with consciousness. In contradistinction to the id, it tends to organisation into a united whole.

Ego-Syntonic—Fitting into the harmony of the ego and thus acceptable by it and helping to integrate it or build it up.

Empathy—A state of sympathetically assuming the feelings of another person and so identifying oneself with him.

Endocrine Glands—Glands which produce internal secretions that enter the blood- or lymph-stream directly.

Endocrinology—The science which is concerned with ductless-gland secretions and the autonomic nervous system.

Endo-Psychic Phantasy—Phantasy having its origin within the psyche, that is, not activated by any external stimulus, somatic or environmental.

Erotic—Sexual.

Extravert, Extrovert—One who turns his interests outward and experiences his emotional life in relation to the stimuli of the external world.

Fetish—Anything which is attractive on account of its association, usually through unconscious elements, with erotic pleasure.

Fixation—Arrest of a portion of the libidinal stream at an immature stage of development, either with reference to its erotogenic zone or with reference to its object attachment or both. The level of a fixation determines the type of any psychosis or psychoneurosis which later may occur, and the nature if its object-attachment may determine its presenting form.

Flagellation—The act of whipping as a sexual excitement.

Frustration—The action of frustrating, or an obstacle or force which stands in the way of gratification of or the aim of an instinct.

Genital Organisation—That mature stage of libidinal development when the component instincts have become synthesised with genital primacy and full capacity for object-love. In infancy it gives rise to the Oedipus complex and in later life to psychosexual union.

Hallucination—A false sensory perception referred to one of the special sense organs as of hearing, sight, smell, etc.

Heterosexuality—Love for or erotic interest in a person of the opposite sex, i.e. normal psychosexual development.

Homosexuality—Sexual desire for a member of the same sex.

Hypnagogic State—A state between sleeping and awakening.

Hypochondria or Hypochondriasis—A condition of morbid anxiety about the health, in which various healthy organs are believed to be diseased.

Hysteria—A psychoneurotic disorder resulting from a conflict between the libido, including non-genital organisation thereof, and the ego or super-ego, in which the libidinal drives are repressed and thus excluded from direct or conscious expression, and in which the unconscious repressed material later, through displacement and conversion, finds an outlet by an indirect somatic pathway and thus produces symptoms. Freud describes two principal varieties: (1) anxiety hysteria, in which the predominating symptom is anxiety but distinguishable from anxiety neurosis in that the aetiological factors are psychological (such as infantile sexual traumata) rather than physical (e.g. disturbances in the current sex life); and (2) conversion hysteria, in which the principal symptoms are physical (hysterical pains, paralyses, etc.). Fixation hysteria is a less important concept applied sometimes to cases where the form or locus of the symptom has been strongly determined by some external factor, e.g. by a wound or physical illness.

Id—The concept of an undifferentiated primitive mind containing only innate urges, instincts, desires and wishes without consciousness or any appreciation of reality, and apparently dominated by the pleasure principle. Unlike the ego it is not organised or integrated, so that contrary and incompatible urges can exist side by side in it without necessarily entering into conflict with each other.

Id Resistance—Resistance to analytical progress emanating from the id, usually due to the energy of the repetitive instinct, or to a disinclination to permit modification of pleasure-giving instinct patterns.

Imago—The fantastic image formed in infancy from an erroneous conception of a loved or hated person.

Infantile Amnesia—Refers to the memory blank which evidently obscures the adult's recollection of certain early periods of his infancy. It does *not* imply its literal meaning of memory blanks occurring *in* infancy.

Inhibition—Restraint or frustration of an impulse by an opposing force, usually by an intra-phychic force. A frustration from within the psyche.

Instincts—Innate patterns of discharge of tension.

Intra-Psychic—Within the mind.

Introjection—A mental process by which one identifies himself with another person or object incorporating it into his ego-system, so that the previous object-cathexis is transferred to a portion of his ego and this brings about a profound change in the intra-psychic libidinal situation. It is a process of assimilation of the object and of feelings associated to it; whereas ' projection ' is a process of dissimilation.

Introversion—The reversal of the libidinal stream from outward-seeking to inward-absorption, with consequent withdrawal of interest from the external world to the internal world of self. When extreme in degree it is one of the characteristics of schizophrenia, melancholia, hypochondriasis, etc.

Inversion (Sexual inversion)—A condition of the sexual instinct being turned to persons in the image of oneself or of one's parent of the same sex as oneself; homosexuality. Havelock Ellis uses the term in a special sense to imply 'inborn' constitutional abnormality towards persons of the same sex. It is thus a narrower term than 'homosexuality, which includes all sexual attractions between persons of the same sex, even when seemingly due to the accidental absence of the natural objects of sexual attraction, a phenomenon of wide occurrence among all human races and among most of the high animals' (Havelock Ellis, *Studies in the Psychology of Sex*, vol. 2, p. 1). 'Inversion' is not generally used in this restricted sense but more commonly as a synonym for homosexuality.

Libidinal Fixation or Libido Fixation—The retention of a portion of the libido at an early level of psychic growth, commonly with special reference to some particular erotogenic zone (e.g. anal-fixation) or to some early object attachment (e.g. mother-fixation).

Libidinal Organisation—The emotional pattern or system of sequences assumed by the libido. The libido passes through many stages in the course of development. From oral to genital the component instincts all have their own organisation or pattern, but full maturity is reached only at the genital level of libidinal organisation with its whole-object (persons as such) relationship.

Libido—The energy of the sexual instinct and of its psychosexual component instincts. It is subject to many vicissitudes. For example, it can become aim-inhibited (i.e. orgasm-inhibited) and undergo unlimited displacement, even on to the person's own ego (narcissism, self-love), asexual objects and abstract ideas.

Masturbation—The act of producing sexual feeling by manual manipulation of one's own genital organ or other erotogenic zone.

Migraine—Sick headache; a symptom complex occurring periodically and characterized by pain in the head usually unilateral, vertigo, nausea and vomiting, and visual symptoms including intolerance of light. In my opinion atypical migraine (i.e. without one or more of the classical symptoms and usually undiagnosed) is responsible for many 'mysterious' aches and pains and visceral disturbances.

Narcissism—Love of oneself.

Neurosis—A functional nervous disorder. By some writers used to designate any psychogenic illness.

Nymphomania—A morbid and uncontrollable heterosexual desire in women.

Obsessional Neurosis—A psychoneurosis characterised by the presence of obsessions which dominate the thought processes and behaviour of the patient. Compulsion neurosis.

Oedipus Complex—As in the play (*Oedipus Rex*) by Sophocles, and as in the Greek legend on which it is founded, the unconscious of man from which these dramatisations originated, has been shown by psychoanalysis to contain a repressed constellation comprising a desire to displace the parent of the same sex and to possess sexually the parent of the opposite sex. It is something infinitely more powerful than common sense that comes into effective conflict with the Oedipus constellation. It is specifically fear of castration which causes total repression of these desires and phantasies. Amongst the evidences of this repression there are the normal horror of incest, intimacy with the very person with whom one had since birth or before birth been most intimate, and the normal tendency to dramatise the repressed constellation in actuality, through the mechanism of displacement, by marrying a person in the image of the repressed imago, and the persistence, at least in physical form, of a repugnance for those in the image of the once hated or displaced parent. Inability to deal adequately in these normal ways with the energy of the repressed complex and consequent regression to fixations at pre-Oedipus levels of libidinal organisation, are the nuclear bases of psychoneurotic, characterological and mental disorders.

Oedipus Fixation—Libidinal fixation to the emotional pattern of the Oedipus complex, with or without change of object.

Oral Erotism—Erotic excitation from stimulation of the mouth or lips, the primary source of erotic feelings in babyhood and continuing in variable degree throughout life in spite of the acquisition of genital maturity with which it becomes associated, as evidenced by the phenomena of kissing and various habits and perversions.

Orgasm—The point at which erotic excitement reaches its acme and becomes involuntary. On the latter account it is suppressed by most persons in proportion to their prevailing anxiety and ill-health.

Orgastic Potency—The degree of capacity to achieve 'perfect' orgasm, that is to say an orgasm which will result in complete reduction of sexual tension and at the same time satisfy the whole psyche, i.e. without residual disturbance or conflict.

Paranoia—A psychosis characterised by systematised delusions commonly of persecution, love or hate. Freud considers that it has its source in repressed (unconscious) homosexual desires.

Parent Surrogate—A substitute for the parent, often not recognised as such.

Part-Objects—Anatomical parts of a person which may be objects of intense love or hate without reference to the person as a whole. For instance, the baby loves the breast or nipple (a part object) without necessarily his mother as a 'whole-object' The persistence of this tendency into adult life is a measure of various libidinal fixations.

Perversion—Any sexual act the object or mechanism of which is both biologically unsound and socially disapproved. Perversions are usually the manifestation of a psychosexual component instinct in substitution for mature genital sexuality.

Phallic—Pertaining to the phallus, the erect penis or its image, worshipped in some religious systems as symbolising generative power in Nature.

Phobia—Morbid or unjustifiable fear, e.g. of some harmless object, activity or situation. It is unconsciously associated with some repressed and feared instinct desire.

Polymorphous Pervert—One who exhibits the pre-genital phases of sexuality, natural in infants, including oral and anal erotism, sadism, exhibitionism, etc.

Pre-Genital Sexuality—The infantile organisation of the sexual pattern in which the component instincts and the pre-genital erotogenic zones, such as oral, anal and phallic, are absorbing the greater part of the libido.

Projection—The attributing to persons or things outside one self of mental processes, affects, etc., that originated within one's own mind (and have been repressed), with relief of tension; common in varying degrees to all minds, with consequent impairment of their reality appreciation. It is very characteristic of paranoia. (Cf. *Introjection*).

Psyche—Mind.

Psychiatry—That branch of medical science which deals with mental diseases and disorders.

Psychogenic—Originating in the mind.

Psychopathology.—The study of morbidity in the psyche.

Psychoneurosis—Psychogenic illness (i.e. without organic cause) characterised by derangement of the normal ways of gratification of the libido due to unconscious conflict, and, while leaving the ego or reason relatively unimpaired (cf. *Psychosis*), giving rise to a variety of symptoms and pathological states which are amenable to psychotherapy.

Psychosis—Insanity. Mental illness which includes the ego or reason and therefore the person's relationship to reality. (Cf. *Psychoneurosis*).

Psychotherapy—The treatment of psychoneurotic, characterological and psychotic disorders by psychological methods, usually one of the forms of mind analysis, or by explanation, persuasion, re-education, relaxation, suggestion, hypnosis, vegetotherapy (Reich) or by occupational therapy.

Rationalisation—The attributing of reasons for judgments, ideas or actions which are otherwise(usually emotionally) determined.

Reaction Formation—A character trait, or its development, unconsciously designed to hold in check, conceal or contradict a tendency of an opposite kind. Thus obsessional cleanliness would be a reaction formation against repressed dirtying tendencies. Disgust, shame and morality are other reaction formations.

Regression—The reversal of the normal direction of the libidinal stream so that early infantile stages of its development (fixation points) are reactivated.

Repression—The rejection from consciousness, by an unconscious mechanism, of mental material, concepts and affects, which are unwelcome. Analysis has shown that this material remains active, and dynamic in the unconscious, that the expenditure of repressing energy continues and that the repressed commonly re-emerges in altered forms such as symptoms.

Resistance—The mental force arrayed against the emergence into consciousness of painful, disagreeable or unwanted material, and which activates the mechanism of repression.

Sadism—The achievement of erotic pleasure by victimising the sexual object, commonly by inflicting helplessness or pain upon him.

Schizophrenia—Split mind. A psychosis, usually in early life, or before middle life, characterised by repressed affect and interest with introversion, dissociation from reality and progressive dementia.

Screen Memories—Memories which by carrying the affects of some earlier experience serve to relieve to some extent the tension of that experience and thereby to cover, or inhibit, its emergence into consciousness.

Scotoma—A blind spot in the mind.

Spasmodic Dysphagia—Difficulty in swallowing, especially in hysteria.

Sublimation—The process of deflecting libido from sexual aims to interests of a non-sexual and socially approved nature.

Super-Ego—That part of the mental apparatus developed in early life by the mechanism of repressing frustrated impulses, such as aggression, and projecting them on the frustrators and subsequently introjecting them. Its function is largely to oppose the id, often unreasonably, and even to criticise and punish the ego if it tends to accept id demands. It is a sort of primitive unconscious conscience.

Symptomatology—The study of symptoms, usually of the specific disease or syndrome under consideration.

Thyrotoxicosis—Poisoning by an excess of thyroid secretion; exophthalmic goiter.

Transference—A displacement of any affect from one person to another. Specifically during analysis the affects originally felt during infancy for the parents become unconsciously displaced on to the person of the analyst so that the analysand feels towards him unjustifiable love and hate and has no insight into the phenomenon and its irrelevance.

Tumescence—A swelling-up. Specifically the turgidity produced in the sexual organs during the pre-orgasm stage of sexual excitement.

Unconscious—A region of the psyche which contains mental processes and constellations which are ordinarily inaccessible to consciousness, commonly owing to the process of repression. The technique of mind analysis is especially designed to bring this unconscious material into consciousness by overcoming the resistances and repressing forces, as it is from the unconscious conflicts or complexes and their opposing forces or reaction formations that all symptoms emanate.

Whole-Object—The person as a whole, in contradistinction to exclusive interest in some anatomical part. (Cf. *Part Objects*).

INDEX

For Product Safety Concerns and Information please contact our EU
representative GPSR@taylorandfrancis.com
Taylor & Francis Verlag GmbH, Kaufingerstraße 24, 80331 München, Germany